Aids to Psychiatry

Aids to Psychiatry

H. G. Morgan
MA, MD (Cantab), FRCP, FRCPsych, DPM (Lond)

Norah Cooke Hurle Professor of Mental Health, University of Bristol;
Honorary Consultant Psychiatrist, South Western
Regional Health Authority

In collaboration with

M. H. Morgan
MA, MD (Cantab), FRCP

Consultant Clinical Neurophysiologist, South Western Regional Health
Authority; Clinical Teacher in Medicine, University of Bristol

SECOND EDITION

CHURCHILL LIVINGSTONE
EDINBURGH LONDON MELBOURNE AND NEW YORK 1984

CHURCHILL LIVINGSTONE
Medical Division of Longman Group UK Limited

Distributed in the United States of America by
Churchill Livingstone Inc., 1560 Broadway, New
York, N.Y. 10036, and by associated companies,
branches and representatives throughout the world.

First edition 1979
Second edition 1984
  Reprinted 1987

ISBN 0 443 02613 0

British Library Cataloguing Publication Data
Morgan, H. G.
    Aid to psychiatry.—2nd ed.
    1. Medicine—Psychiatry
    I. Title   II. Morgan, M.H.
    616.89   RC545

Library of Congress Cataloging in Publication Data
Morgan, H. G. (Howard Gethin)
    Aids to psychiatry.

    Includes index.
    1. Psychiatry.   I. Morgan, M. H. (Margaret Hilary)
II. Title.
RC545.M675   1984   616.89   83-12771

Produced by Longman Singapore Publishers Pte Ltd.
Printed in Singapore

Preface

This book aims to present the essentials of sound examination technique whether in the writing of answers or in the clinical and viva situation. It is not intended as a substitute for wider reading, and regular reference is made to relevant recent review articles.

The approach throughout is to emphasise the marshalling of facts with due regard to their priority and relationship to the realities of clinical practice rather than in an encyclopaedic way. Most important of course is the ability to distinguish essential information from that which is less relevant, particularly with regard to clinical features which are invariable or very common in any condition rather than occasional and infrequent.

A systematic approach to clinical psychiatry and important special topics is followed by consideration of certain aspects of neurology and neurophysiology which the trainee is likely to meet in the clinical situation.

The second edition contains new sections on psychosomatic and affective disorders, drugs and electroconvulsive therapy, as well as on recent developments in mental health legislation.

The final section on examination techniques is meant to be read in parallel with the remainder of the text, dealing as it does with general principles whereby facts and opinions may be marshalled and presented most effectively.

Bristol 1984

H. G. M.
M. H. M.

Contents

Clinical psychiatry

Psychopathology

MENTAL PHENOMENA

THOUGHT PROCESSES

Disordered form
Deviation from rational, logical, goal directed thinking.

Autistic thinking
Directed by inner fantasies associated with social withdrawal. Less subject to correction by reality than is normal thinking.

Blocking
Sudden cessation in the flow of thought or speech; occurs in schizophrenia.

Schizophrenic thought disorder
Disturbance in association leading to subtle discontinuities in the flow of speech (knight's move, derailment). May lead to neologisms (newly invented words), or incoherence when severe.

Pressure of speech
Voluble and difficult to interrupt. Often related to anxiety.

Flight of ideas
High speed, leaps from one subject to another connected tenuously together, and distractible in response to environmental stimuli. Often includes punning. Common in hypomanic illness.

Clang associations
Dictated by chance sounds of words rather than their meanings. Often found with flight of ideas.

Retardation
Slowing of speech as in depression when it may be part of a general picture of psychomotor retardation.

Mutism
Refusal to speak whether for conscious or unconscious reasons.

Disordered content
Obsessions
The pathological presence of a persistent and repetitive thought,
feeling or impulse that cannot be eliminated from consciousness by
any logical effort. On quiet reflection the patient recognises that it
has no rational basis and that it is due to his own psychological
processes rather than some outside influence. Resistance to it is
accompanied by anxiety. In obsessional compulsive neurosis may
lead to severe disturbance in behaviour.

Delusions
A false idea which is held against all evidence to the contrary and
which is out of context with the patient's cultural background. It is
incorrigible and egocentric.

> *Types*
> Paranoid: ideas of persecution and injustice.
> Depressive: morbid guilt, self blame, futility.
> Hypochondriacal: concern with bodily and personal attributes
> and may be bizarre.
> Grandiose: over-estimation of personal qualities, abilities,
> finances (as in hypomanic illness).
> Passivity: abnormal influences on bodily processes by
> outside agencies (as in schizophrenic illness).
> Reference: excessive focus of attention from others, often
> associated with undue sensitivity or paranoid ideation.
> Autochthonous (apophanous): sudden onset, fully elaborated
> apparently not related to situations or current preoccupation
> (in schizophrenia).
> Systematised: usually in chronic schizophrenic psychosis,
> when a rational internal consistency between various
> delusions is developed.

INTELLECTUAL FUNCTION

Level of consciousness
Organic states may lead to confusion in which there is
disorientation in time, place and person, with feelings of
bewilderment. In clouding of consciousness there is similar
disturbance of perception and attention with subsequent amnesia.
When there is also marked anxiety a state of delirium exists and
there may also be hallucinations, paranoid ideation and
consequently overactive or aggressive behaviour.

Coma
Profound loss of consciousness due to organic cause. Deepest levels may be associated with loss of all responses and even reflexes.

Stupor
A state of relative non responsiveness to the environment. May be part of pre coma in organic disturbance. The psychogenic type (depressive or catatonic) associated with full awareness of environment.

Attention
In the normal state this involves a central focus of high intensity with extension to include a variable amount of peripheral material in a less clear way. Both intensity and extent of attention may be impaired by psychological and organic factors, often in a fluctuant way.

Variability is a marked feature of early organic impairment.

Distractibility is common in hypomanic euphoria.

Intense preoccupation with a single theme may occur in depression (guilt) or obsessional states (phobic objects or rituals).

Selective inattention is similar to the defence of denial with avoidance of matters that generate anxiety.

In hypnosis there is restricted awareness with intense focus on one area of consciousness and heightened suggestibility.

Orientation
The ability to recognise one's surroundings and their temporal and spatial relationship to oneself, or to appreciate one's relationship to the environment.

This requires adequacy of exteroceptive data, effective recent memory and correct intellectual adjustment to outer reality (level of consciousness, freedom from delusional thinking).

Concerns
> *Time:*   (hour, day, week and year).
> *Place*:   (present location, its nature, home address, reasons for being in present situation).
> *Person*:   (Identity of self and others).

May be related to organic disorder but psychogenic factors may lead to disorientation as in hysterical dissociation.

Memory

Registration
Impaired by any reduction in consciousness and awareness. Alcohol, drug induced or other organic disorders of the central nervous system. Psychogenic factors include severe anxiety and panic states.

Retention
Extremely rapid decay in 'curve of forgetting' may occur in certain organic brain diseases, e.g. Korsakoff's Psychosis.

Recall
Amnesia is the partial or total inability to recall past experiences. Psychogenic impairment usually related to emotional difficulties, selective for painful events, either recent or distant, and memories may return. In gross hysterical state there may be global amnesia involving all past events and identity. May be associated with physical flight to new and strange surroundings (fugue). Organic amnesia may be irreversible, usually concerns recent events and may leave remote memory intact. Not specifically selective for emotionally traumatic events. Important to note that typical hysterical amnesia may occur in addition to underlying organic brain disorder, and may even be precipitated by it.

Deja vu
Illusion of recognition in which a new situation is incorrectly regarded as a repetition of a previous memory. Common in normal states, anxiety or epileptic aura.

Jamais vu
Illusion of failure to recognise familiar situations.

Confabulation
The filling of gaps in memory by false imagined experiences which the patient believes to be true.

Dysphasia and aphasia
Specific memory disorder for words and language related to organic brain disturbance in the dominant temporal lobe (speech centre), and contiguous areas.

PERCEPTION

The awareness of objects, qualities and relations that follow stimulation of peripheral sensory organs as distinct from awareness that results from memory.

Illusions
Perceptual misinterpretation of a real external sensory experience. Often dictated by dominant affective state, e.g. anxiety which may lead to threatening distortion of visual experiences.

Hallucinations
Apparent perception of an external object when no real corresponding object exists. An internal psychological event is mistakenly attributed to an external source.

Any sensory modality may be involved: may refer to external surroundings or to bodily function.

When caused by organic factors there may be impaired consciousness. Organic causes include hallucinogenic drugs, epilepsy, delirium due to toxic agents or alcohol/barbiturate withdrawal states. Psychogenic causes include schizophrenic psychosis which typically occurs in the setting of clear consciousness. May be hypnogogic (preceding sleep) or hypnopompic (on waking).

AFFECT

The feeling tone that accompanies ideation. Synonymous with emotion. Mood refers to a sustained affective state. Affect may be shallow, inappropriate (does not relate to stimuli or situation) labile, or qualitatively changed as in depression, euphoria, anxiety or anger. Consequent behaviour changes such as aggression may be closely associated with disorders of affect.

Anxiety
An unpleasant emotional state characterised by feelings of apprehension, impending threat or danger. Associated with characteristic pattern of somatic and autonomic changes such as increased sweating, tremor, dry mouth, tachycardia and subjective feelings of tension. May be either free floating, or phobic when it is focussed on specific objects or situations.

Depression
Varies from mild dejection to deep melancholia and despair. Often closely associated with anxiety. When severe there may be secondary disorders of ideation (self blame and futility, hypochondriasis, suicidal thoughts) and of behaviour (retardation, self neglect or agitation when anxiety is also marked).

Euphoria and elation
Elevation of mood with feelings of emotional and physical well being combined with optimism concerning the life situation. When pathological it is usually quite clearly excessive and inappropriate, and may then be accompanied by over-confidence, increased motor activity and impaired judgement.

Ambivalence
The coexistence of opposite emotions and attitudes towards a given object or situation. A common cause of mood swings or oscillation between mild euphoria and depression/anxiety (cyclothymia).

Depersonalisation
A feeling of unreality and strangeness concerning one's own person. May feel outside the self observing it objectively and feeling separate from it. May occur in normals especially with fatigue, or in epilepsy, psychosis (depressive or schizophrenic) or as a hysterical phenomenon.

Derealisation
Loss of sense of reality concerning one's surroundings. Closely associated with depersonalisation. May occur together with severe anxiety in certain phobic states.

GENERAL BEHAVIOUR
Closely related to affective, cognitive and perceptual mental function.

Over-activity
Agitation is a state of restless motor activity that is a manifestation of emotional tension.

Hyperkinesis in children may be related to organic or emotional disturbance.

General increase in activity may be related to euphoric mood states.

Focussed on compulsions and rituals in obsessional compulsive states.

Under-activity
Depressive retardation may lead to slowing of response and ultimate stupor. Psychasthenic states due to anxiety may limit activities because of feelings of fatigue and exhaustion.

Catatonic stupor in schizophrenic patients may lead to prolonged periods of inactivity.

Self neglect
May be related to:
— retardation and ideas of futility in depressive psychosis.
— preoccupation with fantasies and delusions in schizophrenia.
— excitement and lack of judgement in hypomania.
— intellectual impairment in dementia.

Abnormal movements
Stereotypies: the frequent repetition of any speech or action. Common in chronic schizophrenia.

Mannerisms: idiosyncratic elaboration of normal movements, common in chronic schizophrenia.

Echolalia: pathological repetition by imitation of speech of another person. Called echopraxia when this involves imitation of movement.

Cerea flexibilitas: maintenance of imposed posture as in hypnosis or catatonic schizophrenia.

Negativism: resistance to suggestion, tending to do the opposite, as seen in catatonic schizophrenia.

INSIGHT

Full insight requires a correct understanding of the severity, implications and causes of one's illness.

A psychotic patient may not recognise the presence of illness and may fail to accept any such proposition. He may later recover only partial insight accepting that he had previously been ill but remaining unwilling to agree to its psychiatric nature.

Neurotic illness is characterised by insight into the fact of disability, through true awareness of the nature of the underlying psychological factors is often absent.

The chronic brain syndrome (dementia) may lead to severe loss of insight because of impaired judgement secondary to loss of memory and other intellectual abilities. Acute clouding of consciousness also impairs insight.

MENTAL MECHANISMS

Psychoanalytic theory proposes that during development defence strategies are used to mediate between unconscious instinctual drives and the strictures of outside reality.

The repertoire of defences which an individual possesses dictates his character traits.

Defences occur as part of normal development and everyday life: they are not in themselves pathological unless they become excessive or fail to maintain adequate functioning of the individual. Defences may be classified according to the libidinal phase at which they arise, or according to the psychopathology with which they are associated, or whether they are basic or composite.

Repression
Given a central position by Freud. Leads to inability to remember unpleasant wishes or impulses. Common in hysterical, dissociative behaviour but may occur as part of other defences, e.g. sublimation.

Displacement
Shifting of emotion from one idea or object to another in a way that causes less anxiety and guilt.

Reaction formation
An unacceptable impulse is transformed into its opposite. Common in obsessional neurosis.

Isolation
Separation of an idea from the affect which accompanies it.

Undoing
Attempts to cancel out a previously committed act by counter actions. Characteristic of obsessional compulsive states with expiatory rituals which attempt to undo some forbidden act or cancel the effects of a wish to which has been attributed imaginary power of action.

Rationalisation
This provides alternative explanation for instinctual motives and drives.

Intellectualisation
Excessive use of intellectual processes to avoid affective experience.

Denial
May refer to the affect associated with an idea or event or may include the whole episode.

Projection
One's own feelings and wishes are attributed to another person. Common in normals and fundamental in paranoid psychosis.

Regression
A return to an earlier state of psychological development in order to avoid tension and conflict of the present. Common in normals under stress as well as in pathological states.

Counter phobic mechanisms
Attempt to alleviate phobic anxieties by excessive activity in specific relation to the area of concern.

Withdrawal and avoidance
Removal of the self from conflict situations. This may lead to a failure to resolve them.

Introjection
Qualities of a loved object are internalised and the distinction between it and the self tends to be minimised or obliterated. This attempts to reduce painful awareness of separateness and loss.

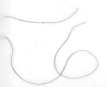

Identification
Usually with a loved object: may also be dictated by guilt.

Acting out
The living out (in action) of warded-off memories when the links between the action and the memory are obscure to the patient.

Sublimation
Important in normals. Psychic energy (often sexual) is deflected to another goal which is more acceptable to the individual concerned.

Organic disorders

A. ENDOCRINE, METABOLIC AND DEFICIENCY DISORDERS

THYROTOXICOSIS

May present with psychological symptoms which are almost invariably present.

Common. Anxiety, hyperactivity, emotional lability. Often no preceding history of anxiety and may be no psychological precipitants.

Less common. Depression with agitation or apathy, early morning waking. May persist after return to euthyroid state, and require antidepressant therapy. Euphoria or 'hypomanic veneer'.

Rare. Acute organic confusion (in severe toxicity), schizophrenic reaction.

MYXOEDEMA

Basically an organic mental syndrome with secondary psychological features depending on personality make up. Most commonly found in the elderly.

Common. Memory impairment, dulled comprehension. May lead to irreversible dementia. Depression with lethargy, irritability (may present in this way): can persist after return to euthyroid state and require antidepressant therapy.

Less common. Coma: may present in this way, often precipitated by infection, high mortality when hypothermia also present. (<35°C). Excessive suspiciousness, paranoid and hallucinatory psychosis. Mania.

VITAMIN B 12 DEFICIENCY

Distinctive. Memory deficits, poor concentration: found in 25% of patients with Addisonian anaemia. May precede neurological and haematological abnormality. Screen for B12 deficiency: all undiagnosed organic brain syndromes, especially in elderly, post gastrectomy, other intestinal diseases, severe chronic dietary deficiency.

Non specific. Affective disorder (anxiety, irritability, depression) in 20%. Folic acid deficiency is said to be more likely to cause affective disorder (56%) (Shorvon et al 1980).

NICOTINIC ACID DEFICIENCY (Pellagra)

Tryptophan deficient diets. Neglect of diet in elderly. Secondary to chronic diarrhoea. Initial depression. Later confusion, delirium and dementia.

HEPATIC ENCEPHALOPATHY

A range of neuropsychiatric disorders associated with hepatic insufficiency.

Clinical features
Chronic organic brain syndrome punctuated by episodic disorders of consciousness, with or without delirium, and finally coma.

In early stages:
— exaggeration of personality traits
— anxiety, depression or denial
— reversal of sleep rhythm
— slowing of EEG
— fluctuating degrees of concentration, awareness
— constructional apraxia

In later stages:
— confusion, inappropriate behaviour
— delusional ideas, hallucinations
— visual illusions (micropsia)
— hepatic coma (may be heralded by stupor, fits, flapping tremor of hands, hypertonia and hyper-reflexia, extensor plantar responses)

Causes
Due to metabolic changes secondary to liver cell failure. Precise metabolites involved uncertain:
— raised blood ammonia usually found but its level does not correlate closely with severity of symptoms
— toxic products of protein breakdown (such as methionine

and tryptophan metabolites) entering systemic blood supply via new collateral extrahepatic and intrahepatic shunts
— short chain fatty acids may also be toxic
— accumulation of neurotransmitters originating from bacterial protein breakdown in gut
— coma may be precipitated by diuretics, high protein intake, presence of blood in gut, intercurrent infection, sedatives, phonothiazines, monoamine oxidase inhibitors and other antidepressants. Portal systemic shunt (especially if surgically induced in treatment of portal hypertension) may be cause of delusional hallucinatory symptoms and central nervous damage (paraplegia, cerebellar and basal ganglion disease, epileptic fits).

Differential diagnosis
Important to distinguish alcoholic delirium tremens from hepatic encephalopathy if only because sedatives can be fatal in latter.

Liver failure	DTs
Hypoactive apathetic state	Physically overactive
May resemble depression	Vivid visual hallucinations
Irregular flapping tremor may occur	Tremor coarse, rhythmic
EEG: progressive slowing with high amplitude triphasic waves	

CUSHING'S DISEASE

Due to excess production of cortisol with variable amount of adrenal androgens. Adenoma or carcinoma of adrenal cortex 20% adrenal hyperplasia 80%. Psychological symptoms in >50%: more likely when history of previous psychiatric difficulties, improve with adequate treatment of endocrine disorder.

Common. Depression with anxiety or retardation, excessive fatigue, stupor, episodic acute excitement, anxiety, impotence, amenorrhoea, loss of libido. Severity of depression not related to levels of circulating cortisol: it may be rapidly relieved when tumour or hyperplastic gland removed. Tumour less commonly associated with psychiatric symptoms than is hyperplasia.

Less common. Paranoid delusions, auditory hallucinations. Elation, euphoria (2%). Acute organic reactions: may be subjective complaint of memory impairment when objective findings minimal.

ADDISON'S DISEASE

Chronic adrenocortical insufficiency of cortisol, aldosterone, corticosterone and androgens. Primary atrophy (up to 50%). In the past tuberculosis more common. Psychological symptoms present in all severe cases. Mild memory impairment (75%). Organic type symptoms vary with severity of underlying endocrine deficiency and hypoglycaemia: in crisis there may be delirium. Depression (25%), apathy (25%), irritability (up to 50%). Rare to see other psychotic symptoms.

ACTH AND CORTICOSTEROID THERAPY

Psychological symptoms more likely with high doses or prolonged treatment, or history of previous psychiatric difficulties. Euphoria (up to 70%). Depression far less common (contrast Cushing's Disease). Irritability, tension. Psychosis (5%): mania, depression, stupor, disorientation, delusions, hallucinations, catatonia. Psychological dependence with depression as a result of steroid withdrawal sometimes occurs.

HYPOPITUITARISM

Chronic anterior pituitary failure. Most commonly due to post partum ischaemic necrosis. Early loss of libido, pubic and axillary hair. Skin pale, wrinkled. Weight loss not a significant feature. Depression, apathy, self neglect. Sensitivity to cold. Sleepy. Memory impairment. Episodes of confusion, delirium, liability to become comatose and die in absence of endocrine replacement.

FURTHER READING

Beaumont, P. J. V. (1972) Endocrines and psychiatry. *Brit. J. Hosp. Med.,* **April**, 485–497.
Cohen, S. I. (1980). Cushing's syndrome: a psychiatric study of 29 patients. *Brit. J. Psychiat.,* **136**, 120–124.
Michael, R. P., & Gibbons I. K. (1963) Endocrines and neuropsychiatry. *Int. Rev. Neurobiology,* **5**, 243–302.
Shorvon, S. D. et al. (1980). The neuropsychiatry of megaloblastic anaemia. *Brit. Med. J.,* **281**, 1036–1038.

RENAL ENCEPHALOPATHY

Clinical features

May be due to
- — uraemia
- — underlying disease process
- — secondary physical and psychological complications

Uraemic encephalopathy
Essentially an organic brain syndrome. Psychological disturbance
found in 75% of patients who have blood urea of more than 250
mg%. At first: fatigue, headache, poor concentration. Later:
episodic confusion or delirium, coma.

Neurological disorder
Myoclonic jerks, asterixis, (metabolic flap) usually at times of
clouded consciousness, extrapyramidal rigidity, involuntary
movements, neuropathy (painful paraesthesiae, restless legs
syndrome), polymyositis (proximal limb weakness), epileptic fits
(33%), reversible amaurosis.

EEG changes
Diffuse slowing, lowered voltage, episodic epileptic type features.

Psychological disturbance
Depression: early features of uraemia may mimic this, but may
develop secondarily.
Anxiety
Secondary defence mechanisms

Aetiology

Neuropathological. Some neuronal degeneration and loss. May be
overshadowed by vascular complications due to secondary
disorders such as hypertension. Urea itself not neurotoxic.

Electrolyte and acid/base changes. Especially when these are rapid.

Water intoxication

Abnormal neurotransmitter metabolism

Wernicke's encephalopathy: thiamine deficiency.

Iatrogenic. High doses of penicillin may cause fits. Diuretics may
cause hypokalaemia. Immunosupressants and steroids may
predispose to viral or fungal meningoencephalitis or
reticulo-endothetical tumours.

Effects of dialysis
When carried out rapidly or there is severe initial metabolic abnormality, then dialysis may lead to a 'disequilibrium syndrome' of headache, confusion, fits, coma. This may be due to cerebral oedema, or reactive hypoglycaemia may also be a factor.

Dementia may also complicate dialysis. Usually progressive and fatal in few months, often with osteomalacia, multiple bone fractures, orofacial grimacing and fits. Appears to be unrelated to biochemical disturbance, and not improved by further dialysis. May be due to accumulation in brain of aluminium derived from water used in dialysis.

Hospital ward regimes
May involve social isolation and sensory deprivation. These may heighten anxiety, accentuate confusion, precipitate delirium or paranoid reaction.

Renal transplantation donors
Careful psychological screening of potential donors.
Sudden irrational decision suspect especially when family coercion present.
Exclude donor who has markedly ambivalent relationship with recipient.

B. ORGANIC BRAIN SYNDROMES

CHARACTERISTIC CLINICAL FEATURES

Tend to show marked fluctuation in severity, worse at night.
  1. Memory loss (most severe for recent events).
  2. Impairment of consciousness (especially in acute forms).
  3. Disorientation (time, place, person).
  4. Intellectual impairment (defect of grasp, reasoning, social disinhibition).
  5. Non-specific: hallucinations (especially visual) mood disturbances (lability, depression) delusional ideas, focal neurological signs.

ACUTE ORGANIC BRAIN SYNDROME

Disorientation and clouding of consciousness predominate. May also be anxiety, bewilderment, illusions, hallucinations (delirium).

Causes
Metabolic, infective, toxic, traumatic, degenerative, vascular.
  Alcohol or barbiturates withdrawal in habituated individuals, nutritional deficiency (thiamine: external ophthalmoplegia, ptosis).

CHRONIC ORGANIC BRAIN SYNDROME

The dementias
Disorders of recent memory and intellectual impairment
predominate. May be episodic confusion or delirium.
Secondary behavioural disorders.

Senile dementia
After 65 years of age. Particularly common in those aged 75 + .10%
of persons over 65 years suffer from dementia. Size of problem
likely to get bigger due to rise in 75+ population. Increasing
restriction of interests, living in the past, confused wandering at
night common.

Causes
Accentuation of normal ageing with loss of neuronal tissue
(cerebral atrophy).
   Cerebral arteriosclerosis, trauma (cerebral injury, subdural
haematoma), myxoedema, B12 deficiency.

Presenile dementia
Alzheimer's disease. Common. Idiopathic atrophy. Early memory
loss, dressing apraxia, disorientation, fits, extrapyramidal signs.
Neuronal loss, argentophil plaques, neurofibrillary cell changes.
Marked involvement of parietal lobe.

Low pressure hydrocephalus. (Adams syndrome). Ataxia and
urinary incontinence common.

Traumatic. Degree of dementia correlates well with duration of post
traumatic amnesia (duration after injury before continuous memory
recall is established).

Punch-drunk syndrome. Onset many years after stopped boxing.
Dementia, rage reaction, morbid jealousy, impotence, intention
tremor, pyramidal and extrapyramidal signs.

Infective. Neurosyphilis: (General paralysis of the insane; G.P.I.;
tabo-paresis). May present with depression, grandiose paranoid
psychosis (10%), social disinhibition.

Vascular. Cerebral arteriosclerosis: common and may be merely
coincidental with dementia from other cause. Depression often
marked initially.

Metabolic. Hypothyroidism (when chronic and severe).
Hypoglycaemia (intermittent disordered behaviour, confusion or
loss of consciousness).

Chronic renal dialysis. Due to accumulation in brain of aluminium from dialysis fluid.

Anoxic. Coal gas poisoning: beware late deterioration after 10 days.

Genetic. Huntington's chorea. Dominant autosomal gene. Incidence 5/100,000. Some sporadic cases occur (mutation). Onset 30–50 years of age. May be depression or paranoid state initially. Increased family incidence of suicide, antisocial behaviour. All children of an affected parent have 50% chance of developing disease.

Pick's disease. Mendelian dominant. Rare. Early social disinhibition (frontal lobe involvement). Rigid egocentric attitude. Focal neurological deficits common e.g. dysphasia. Memory loss late. Cerebral atrophy, neuronal loss, presence of balloon-like Pick cells.

Neurological disorders. In multiple sclerosis euphoria suggests dementia. Cerebral tumour (disinhibited behaviour when frontal lobe involved).

DIFFERENTIAL DIAGNOSIS OF DEMENTIA

Depression: may present with complaint of poor concentration and memory. Schizophrenia: simulates dementia through autistic behaviour, self neglect. Hysterical amnesia: global or selective for traumatic events. Chronic drug intoxication: slow, poor concentration (may occur in epileptics).

In as many as 31% of patients given a diagnosis of senile dementia this is incorrect: they are in fact suffering from depressive illness or acute confusional state (Ron 1979).

INVESTIGATION OF DEMENTIA

Diagnostic tests relevant to all of the above specified conditions: EMI Scan. Angiography, (subdural haematoma, tumour). Pneumoencephalography.

THE AMNESIC SYNDROME (Korsakow psychosis)

Recent memory defect (can register memory but only minimal recall present). May confabulate, confuse temporal sequence of events. Chronic alcoholism and peripheral neuropathy commonly associated.

Causes. Thiamine deficiency (Wernicke's encephalopathy). Cerebral anoxia, III ventricle tumours. Bilateral medial temporal lobe resection.

Degenerative changes in mid and hind brain, most severe in mammillary bodies and hippocampus.

FURTHER READING

Corsellis, J. A. N. (1969) The pathology of dementia. *Brit. J. Hosp. Med.*, March 695–703.
Kiloh, L. G. (1975) Psychiatric disturbances of organic origin. *Medicine*, **10**, 460–468.
Robertson, E. E. (1978) Organic disorders. In *Companion to Psychiatric Studies.* Ed. Forrest, A., Edinburgh: Churchill Livingstone.
Ron, M. A. et al. (1979) Diagnostic accuracy in presenile dementia. *Brit. J. Psychiat.*, **134**, 161–168.

C. POST OPERATIVE PSYCHOSES

INCIDENCE

1 : 1600 surgical operations (severe enough to require psychiatric admission). Increased risk following:
>   hysterectomy
>   open heart surgery
>   cholecystectomy
>   eye operations.

CAUSES

Metabolic disturbance. Emotional reaction to operation (may be paramount). Withdrawal delirium in alcohol or barbiturate dependent individuals.

CLINICAL VARIANTS

Acute confusional states (when organic factors predominate). Anxiety, depressive or manic states. Schizophrenic psychosis (especially paranoid type).

D· PUERPERAL PSYCHOSES

Psychotic illness developing within six months after childbirth.

INCIDENCE

2–3 per 1000 pregnancies. Recurrence rate 20 per 100 subsequent pregnancies.

CAUSES

Usually multifactorial (metabolic and emotional). More common in elderly primiparae, unmarried, previous psychiatric illness or difficult pregnancies.

CLINICAL FEATURES

As for post operative psychoses. Commences on third or fourth day after delivery. Initial organic confusional fluctuating disturbance. Later more clearly affective (68%) schizophrenic (27%) or organic (4.5%). May be mixed picture. Outcome tends to be better when affective symptoms predominate. Risk of infanticide high in depressive variants.

TREATMENT

Avoid separation if possible (Mother and baby unit). May need physical treatment (phenothiazines and ECT).

FURTHER READING

Paffenberger, R. S. (1964) Parapartum mental illness. *Brit J. Prev. Soc. Med.*, **18**, 189.
Protheroe, C. (1969) Puerperal psychosis. *Brit. J. Psychiat.*, **115**, 9–30.
Seager, C. P. (1960) Post partum mental illness. *J. Ment. Sci.*, **106**, 214.

E. PSYCHIATRIC ASPECTS OF EPILEPSY

ICTAL

Clouding of consciousness a necessary diagnostic feature.

Prodromal
Irritability, tension, restlessness.

Aura
Last few seconds, maximum 1 minute. Stereotyped and compelling. Hallucinations, mood changes, delusional ideas. Rising epigastric sensation may be confused with anxiety.

Seizures
Automatism, particularly in temporal lobe epilepsy (TLE). Behavioural change due to partial fits. Violence rare.

POSTICTAL

Automatism.
Confusional psychosis:
    — may be preceded by series of fits
    — vivid hallucinations
    — delusional ideas (paranoid, religious)
    — may be aggressive if handled tactlessly.

INTERICTAL

Bias in patient selection a major problem in assessing incidence of various disorders.
    No evidence for a specific epileptic personality. Increased risk of psychological difficulties in major epilepsy and TLE. Reflects site and extent of any associated brain damage and previous psychosocial history. Most common when frontal lobes, III ventricular areas involved. Perseverative/paranoid personality in diffuse brain damage, bitemporal epilepsy.

Aggressive behaviour. No adequate control study of epileptics compared with general population.
    Prevalence of epilepsy in prison population 7.1/1000 (general population 4.2/1000).
    Violence not more common in epileptic compared with other prisoners.
    In post traumatic epilepsy, frontal lobe damage predisposes to aggression and criminality.
    Early onset dominant temporal lobe lesion associated with aggressivity (poor social learning).

Depression. Always a serious matter. Often marked variability — may be inverse relation to fit frequency. Especially common in non-dominant temporal lobe lesions.

Suicide. Increased incidence. Access to drugs relevant. Up to 7% life expectancy of suicide in organic brain disorder with epilepsy.

Dementia. No clear evidence that epilepsy *per se* causes dementia. If present likely to be due to concomitant organic cerebral disease. Mimicked by barbiturate over-medication. Prolonged petit mal in childhood (impairs learning).

Chronic schizophreniform psychosis. Rare. May show any cardinal symptom of schizophrenia. Often begins long after onset of epilepsy (median interval 14 years). 65% of cases have TLE.

May be due to organic temporal lobe lesions (particularly dominant side). Association between TLE and psychosis regarded by some as artefact due to patient selection.

Sexual deviation. TLE associated with wide variety of deviant sexual behaviour (hyposexuality, transvestism, fetishism, homosexuality). Especially when temporal lobe lesion occurs initially in infancy.

EPILEPSY AND AUTOMATISM

State of clouded consciousness during or immediately after seizure. Retains control of posture. Performs simple or complex movements/actions. Impaired awareness. May be preceding aura (only in TLE). Periamygdaloid region most common initiating area.

CAUSES

1. TLE
Spike foci in one or both temporal lobes (90%).
Mesial temporal lobe sclerosis (50%).
Aura: abdominal sensations, illusions, hallucinations (especially olfactory), masticatory and tonic movements.

2. Lesions in frontal, parietal, mesial (cingulate) and uncal areas

3. Prolonged petit mal

CLINICAL FEATURES

Last 5 minutes or less in 80%. Never more than 1 hour.
   Initial (impairment) staring, slumping, dazed.
   Midpoint (repetitive) smacking lips, chewing, mumbling, blinking.
   Terminal (integrated) confusion, wandering, paranoid ideas, violence rare (<1%).

DIAGNOSTIC POINTERS

Diagnosis must be based primarily on clinical grounds, but prolonged ambulatory EEG monitoring can be very useful.
Sudden onset, up to few minutes in duration. Unequivocal previous history of epilepsy. Witness may notice impaired awareness. No retrograde amnesia. If offence committed it is unpremeditated and no attempt made to conceal.

DIFFERENTIAL DIAGNOSIS

Hysterical Amnesia and Fugue
Often life crisis with purposeful escape.
Awareness unimpaired during episode.
Amnesia may last hours or weeks.

Malingering
Gross variability and inconsistency.

Stress reaction
Episodic aggressive behaviour under stress.
May last few hours. Inhibited individuals who use denial
mechanisms.
No clinical evidence of epilepsy.
May be histrionic or depressive element.
Rare to injure persons.

Catatonic schizophrenia
Clear consciousness. Episodic aggressive outbursts.
Posturing and sterotyped movements.

Alcohol, drug intoxication

Organic confusion
Hypoglycaemia, infection, cerebral ischaemia, dementia.

Sleep walking
In deep (Stage IV) sleep.
Rare to see repetitive stereotyped behaviour.
Behaviour usually well integrated.
May need sleep EEG to differentiate from epilepsy.

FURTHER READING

Betts, T. A., Merskey, H. & Pond, D. A. (1976) Psychiatry. In *A Textbook of Epilepsy*. Ed. Laidlaw & Richards. Edinburgh: Churchill Livingstone.
Fenton, G. W. (1972) Automatism. *Brit. J. Hosp. Med.*, January 57–64.
Flor. Henry P. (1976) Epilepsy and psychopathology. In *Recent Advances in Clinical Psychiatry 2*. Ed. Granville-Grosman, K. pp. 263–295. Edinburgh: Churchill Livingstone (Review).
Stevens, J. (1975) Interictal phenomena. In *Advances in Neurology, Vol. 11*, 85–112.

Psychosomatic disorders

A. OBESITY

ARBITRARY DEFINITION

When body weight exceeds 120% ideal weight for sex, height, medium frame.

PREVALENCE

More common in females, middle age, lower social class.
Females in London:
— age 40–49 years: 30% } are obese
— social class IV–V: 50% }
Children in Buckinghamshire (14-year-olds):
— girls 32.4% } are obese
— boys 3.6% }

CLINICAL FEATURES

Untreated obese individuals show few neurotic traits.
Obese patients have increased incidence of emotional difficulties.
Social stereotype leads to scapegoating and exclusion especially in childhood. Predisposes to denial, self loathing and over-estimate of body size.

NEUROLOGICAL SUBSTRATE

Energy homeostasis achieved by balance between ventromedial and lateral hypothalamic nuclei (hunger and satiety centres). These under influence of internal cues (metabolic) and external cues (palatability of foods, learnt attitude to food).

CAUSES

Predisposing
Psychological factors less obvious in late onset type.
Genetic. MZ twins high concordance for body weight.

Developmental. Increased total fat cell number through overfeeding in childhood. Aberrant family attitudes to food: substitute for comfort, obesity equated with well-being.

Precipitating
Emotional upset may lead to obesity in predisposed individuals because eating causes tension release.

TREATMENT

High default and relapse rate, variable motivation.
1. *Diet.* Dietary (calorie) restriction over extended period.
2. *Psychological.* Extended individual/group support. Dieting may lead to irritability, depression, loss of denial defence. Conjoint therapy with spouse (deal with factors preventing dieting in family situation).
3. *Drugs.* Anorectics: use intermittently (danger of dependence). Phentermine and chlorphentermine useful in lethargic depressed patients. Fenfluramine a central anorectic with peripheral effect on glucose uptake. May lead to depression on withdrawal. Useful in the anxious and overactive.
4. *Surgical adjuncts.* Jaw wiring: useful in initiating weight loss when all else fails.
   Ileojejujonostomy: increased assertiveness and sexual interest. Family adjustment difficulties may follow. May be up to 25% incidence of post-operative depression and suicidal ideas.

FURTHER READING

Colley, J. R. T. (1974) Obesity in schoolchildren. *Brit. J. Prev. Soc. Med.,* **28,** 221–225.
Kalucy, R. S. (1977) Obesity. In *Modern Trends in Psychosomatic Medicine,* **3,** 404–429.
Silverstone, J. T. (1968) Psychosocial aspects of obesity. *Proc. Roy. Soc. Med.,* **61,** 371.
Silverstone, J. T. (1973) Psychological and social aspects of obesity. In *Brit. J. Hosp. Med.,* July 39–42.

B. ANOREXIA NERVOSA

Females outnumber males 15:1 (Case register data).
Most common in upper social classes.
Age onset 15.5 years average (87% within 5 years of menarche).
Point prevalence: 1% girls age 16–18 years in private schools.
1–2% of female university students.
Minor variants in community more common than severe cases.
Recent increased incidence likely, especially in less severe form.

CLINICAL FEATURES

1. Physical
Marked loss of body weight and malnutrition due to:
— purposive avoidance of 'fattening foods', self induced
  vomiting
— and purgation, excessive exercise, subterfuges in disposal of
  food.
Nutritional myopathy (gross muscle wasting with good power).
Bradycardia, peripheral cyanosis, normal secondary sexual hair,
episodic bulimia.

2. Endocrine
Specific hypothalamic-hypophyseal failure of gonadotrophin
secretion.

In female: Amenorrhoea precedes or coincident with weight loss in
50%.
In males: Loss of sexual interest, impotence.

Low oestrogen, testosterone, gonadotrophin. Euthyroid. Raised
G.H. and cortisol. Delayed return of cyclical gonadotrophin output
from pituitary when weight returns to normal.

3. Psychological
a. *Marked fear of becoming fat: explicit or implicit in behaviour.*
   Strives to be thin, believes self to be fat when thin; loss of
   judgement in food needed, sets weight limits.
b. *Non-specific.*
   Depression 25–50%, obsessional symptoms 20–25%, anxiety
   40%.
   Highly conscientious, strives to achieve.

CAUSES AND PSYCHODYNAMICS

The psychobiological regression hypothesis suggests that anorexia
nervosa is a state of regression (triggered by nutritional
deprivation) which then allows phobic avoidance of personal
conflict. Puberty is a weight-related event, signalled by the passing
of a threshold body weight: patients with anorexia nervosa have a
neuroendocrine state which resembles pre-puberty. Loss of weight
may be rewarding and liable to lead to anorexia nervosa in certain
vulnerable adolescents (those who are experiencing difficulties
with the transitions inherent in adolescence), because the biological
regression which it brings leads also to psychological regression
with temporary relief from conflicts over such matters as sexuality
(loss of libido) or emancipation (invalidism). This process of
'switching off' tends to be self perpetuating because the individual
fears weight gain with return of conflicts. Deliberate dieting

(common in adolescent females) is therefore at risk of precipitating anorexia nervosa in a small proportion of vulnerable individuals who embark upon it. Early menarche may similarly act as precipitant. Family factors may be important: high incidence of marital difficulties in parents and psychiatric illness in mother: high parental expectation to achieve (themselves and children).

DIFFERENTIAL DIAGNOSIS

Malabsorption syndrome, Crohn's disease, reticulosis, diabetes mellitus, thyrotoxicosis, gastro intestinal neoplasia.

Depressive illness, phobic anxiety state, obsessional neurosis, paranoid psychosis (with fears of food being poisoned).

Bulimia nervosa characterised by intractable urges to overeat (often leading to 'binge' episodes of massive food intake), use of self-induced vomiting and/or purgatives to avoid the fattening effects of food. There is also a characteristic fear of becoming fat. Bulimia nervosa may be unsuspected because body weight is often near normal. It may be much more common than anorexia nervosa (although 35–50% of patients with bulimia nervosa go through a state which is identical with anorexia nervosa). Note also anorexia nervosa is complicated by binge eating in up to 50% of cases.

COMPLICATIONS

Physical
Oedema, impaired excretion of water load (especially in chronic illness). Electrolyte disturbance, e.g. hypokalemia, alkalosis when vomiting. Dehydration. Secondary hyperaldosteronism. Hypercholesterolaemia. Carotenaemia. Hypoglycaemia. Hypothermia. Moderate normochromic normocytic anaemia Hb. 10–11 G%. (Occasionally aplastic crisis.)
Follicular hyperkeratosis. Lanugo type hair on trunk.

Psychological
Intense family reaction (anxiety, hostility, wish to control). Aversion to food worse when weight loss severe. Reactive depression and suicide risk.

TREATMENT

Initial
Restoration of normal nutrition (may be urgent). Admit to hospital when body weight falling progressively and has reached 60% normal average body weight or less.

Psychotherapy
Ongoing support, help to face precipitating factors.

Drugs and physical
Anxiolytics and antidepressants when symptomatically indicated.
(High doses of chlorpromazine recommended by some.)

LONG TERM OUTCOME

Good (normal weight and menstruation) 40%. Intermediate 27%.
Poor (constant low weight and amenorrhoea) 29%. Death 5%.
Body weight has to be maintained near normal for some time
before menstruation returns.

PROGNOSTIC FACTORS

Poor outcome when illness prolonged, onset in late teens or older,
childhood adjustment difficulties, poor relationship with family and
with other children in school.

FURTHER READING

Crisp, A. H. (1970) *Modern Trends in Psychosomatic Medicine*, **2**, 124–147.
Crisp, A. H. (1978) Anorexia Nervosa. *Medicine 11*, 537–542.
Fairburn, C. (1982) Binge-eating and bulimia nervosa. Smith Kline & French
    publications. Vol 1 No. 4.
Hill, O. W. (1977) *Modern Trends in Psychosomatic Medicine*, **3**, 382–404.
Palmer, R. L. (1980) Anorexia nervosa. Harmondsworth: Penguin Books
Russell, G. F. M. (1970) *Modern Trends in Psychological Medicine*, **2**,
    130–164.
Russell, G. F. M. (1979) Bulimia nervosa: an ominous variant of anorexia
    nervosa. *Psych. Med.*, 9 429–448.
Morgan, H. G. (1982) Anorexia nervosa. *Practitioner*, **226**, 1941–1947

C. ASSESSMENT OF PAIN

DEFINITION

Pain is an unpleasant experience which we primarily associate with
tissue damage, or describe in terms of such damage or both
(Merskey).

PAIN OF PSYCHOLOGICAL ORIGIN

May be: 1. Continuous for long periods by day.
         2. Tends not to be the subject of sharp accentuation.
         3. Is often recognised by patients as having emotional
            precipitants.
         4. May prevent getting off to sleep but not cause
            wakening.

PSYCHOLOGICAL MECHANISMS
1. Influence severity and character of pain due to organic disorder.
2. May perpetuate pain when organic cause has resolved.
3. Can produce pain in absence of organic disease.
    Those which influence pain perception include:
Aggression (arousal and distraction): reduction of pain sensation (battle injuries).
Anxiety/depression: increased pain perception. May present as 'pain problem'.
Schizophrenia: delusional ideas of passivity or bizarre hypochondriasis.
Hysterical conversion.
Malingering.
Identification: bereavement or commonly some painful illness in relative.

ASSESSMENT OF PAIN PROBLEM

(When organic disease is judged absent or trivial).
    Both organic and psychological factors may be present. Need to interview several informants. Aim to get consistent positive psychological evidence from several sources.

Family. Ethnic variation in attitudes, bereavement, current illness, wife pregnant (Couvade syndrome).

Previous personality. Attitudes to illness and tolerance of painful conditions. Hypochondriasis. Mood variation. Situational vulnerabilities.

Previous psychiatric illness. May resemble current symptoms in quality, cause, course.

Life situation. Recent stress, especially those to which vulnerable. Litigation.

The symptoms. Bizarre quality not necessarily indicative of psychogenic cause.

TREATMENT

Beware of escalation in use of sedatives and analgesics. Patients with psychogenic pain often hostile to psychological approach.

FURTHER READING

Merskey, H. and Spear, F. G. (1967) *Pain: Psychological and Psychiatric Aspects*. London: Bailliere Tindell.
Merskey, H. (1975) Pain. *Medicine*, **10**, 424–429.
Stengel, E. (1965) Pain and the psychiatrist. *Brit J. Psychiat.*, **111**, 795–802.

D. ISCHAEMIC HEART DISEASE (IHD)

Behavioural types

A proposed causal link between psychosocial factors and IHD. Implies that inappropriate emotional reaction to stress predisposes to IHD.

Type A characteristics: impatience, sense of urgency, competitiveness, aggressiveness, hyperalertness, explosive speech, abruptness of gesture.
Type B characteristics: the absence of these behavioural features.

Causal mechanisms

Increased incidence of IHD in Type A men (cross sectional and longitudinal studies). Causal factors may involve more rapid blood clotting, increased platelet aggregation in Type A individuals (no difference in serum cholesterol, blood pressure or cigarette smoking).

The twentieth century 'epidemic' of IHD may be due to increased prevalence of Type A behaviour (Rosenman), but other complex aetiological factors also likely.

Risk in Type A is twice that in Type B.

Type A behaviour may be most useful in predicting high risk when combined with other risk factors: when present with hypertension the risk of IHD may be 6% over 2½ years.

Conversely, Type B individuals with low serum lipids and lipoproteins may constitute a low risk group.

Psychological Aspects of Acute IHD

Distress and disability may be more related to psychological and social problems than to organic symptoms themselves.

Concomitants

About 50% of IHD patients have high levels of anxiety and/or depression in between acute episodes of illness, and emotional precipitants of angina include anger, excitement or anxiety (Mayou).

Denial is a significant defence mechanism in 60% of IHD patients: in some it may interfere with management by reducing treatment compliance.

Secondary disability
Irritability
Secondary family problems in 70%. Relatives anxious, overprotective or resentful, avoidance of sexual relationship.
Only a minority discontinue *alcohol intake, smoking.*
Return to work less common in those who had previous personality difficulties and such patients exhibit greater emotional upset during acute IHD. Patients with mild angina tend to remain off work longer than those with severe IHD.

Management
Planned integrated team approach allows effective and prompt attention to be paid to physical, psychological and social factors concurrently.

Emotional wellbeing closely related to adequate reassurance, explanation, management of defence reactions, control of affective disturbance both in patient and relatives.

FURTHER READING

'Type A behaviour and ischaemic heart disease': Editorial. Psychological Medicine (1980), **10**, 603–608.
Mayou, R. (1973) The patient with angina. *Postgrad. Med. J.*, **49**, 250–254.

The psychoses

A. THE SCHIZOPHRENIAS

Emil Kraepelin (1896). Dementia praecox implied deterioration during course of illness. Grouped under this rubric-catatonic, hebephrenic and paranoid states.

Eugene Bleuler (1911). Fundamental disorder involved splitting of psychological functions. Coined term 'schizophrenias': deterioration not inevitable, the content and meaning of psychotic symptoms were emphasised.

Adolf Meyer (1910). Psychobiological school. Saw schizophrenia as a reaction to traumatic life situation. Insisted on unique, idiosyncratic response in each individual, and eschewed general rules of psychodynamics.

1. PHENOMENOLOGY

Delusions
Present in 71%

Primary (autochthonous): not understandable in terms of preceding morbid experience. Sudden onset. Delusional perception when abnormal significance is attached to normal perception which is accorded a sense of urgent importance. Often self referring.

Secondary: arise out of some other morbid experience e.g. persecutory delusions relating to hallucinations.

Delusions may be related to morbid ideas of passivity (influence or control by an outside agency) e.g. thought insertion or withdrawal, or being made to think. Distinguish from 'as if' experiences which lack delusional conviction.

Thought disorder
Low consistency between constructs (Kelly Repertory Grid).
Over-inclusive, asyndetic, imprecise, interpenetrating themes (Cameron).
Concrete thinking, impaired abstract thought (Goldstein).

Hallucinations
Form: auditory 95%, visual 30%, less commonly olfactory, tactile, bodily, gustatory.
Content: usually voices of relatives or other familiar figures. Threatening in 33%.

Schneider's first rank symptoms
Can be reliably detected and defined clearly. Present in 28–72%.

Claimed to be diagnostic when one or more present, in absence of organic brain disease or other relevant pathology. Important to remember that their significance can only be assessed in the light of the total clinical picture, previous personality and cultural background. Great caution in assessment when severe depression or manic elevation of mood present.

The first rank symptoms are:
a. Audible thoughts.
b. Voices arguing, running commentary on patient's actions.
c. Somatic passivity: experiences of physical interference by outside influences.
d. Thought withdrawal, insertion or interruption by outside influence.
e. Thought broadcasting, or believe others to think the same thoughts.
f. Delusional perception.
g. Feelings, impulses, volitional acts thought to be due to others.

First rank symptoms have no theoretical value and have poor prognostic significance. May occur in 13% of mania, 15% depressive disorders, 2% neuroses. Variation in assessment of specificity and validity may be due to inadequate interview method. Careful and extended clinical interview required, based on phenomenological technique, in order to demonstrate first rank symptoms reliably.

Bleuler's fundamental symptoms
Loosened associations between psychological functions, autism, ambivalence, disorders of affect.

These are not easy to detect in a reliable way.

Variation in diagnostic fashion
Concept of schizophrenia is wider in the U.S.A., where in some parts (New York) it is diagnosed twice as often as in Europe.

Incidence
Illness expectancy 15–45 years = 0.5–1%.
First admissions to hospital 15–20/100 000 per annum.

Clinical types

Hebephrenic: *onset* 15–25 years. Thought disorder, incongruous
affect.

Catatonic: 15–40 years. Motor disorders. ? Becoming less
common.

Paranoid: 15–60 years. Delusional ideas (with or without
hallucinations).

Simple: Young adult. Loss of drive, social deterioration.
Dubious entity.

Good prognostic indicators

Acute onset, obvious precipitating stress.
Good previous personality, strong affective component.
Described by Langfeldt (1939) as schizophreniform psychoses.
Well-preserved affect, paranoid (less likely to deteriorate).

Poor prognostic indicators

Onset before 20 years, schizoid previous personality, insidious
onset, hebephrenic type, family history of deteriorating
schizophrenia. This type of clinical picture has been termed
'nuclear' or 'process' type.

2. CLINICAL COURSE

Five years follow-up period (Wing)
Chronic: symptoms throughout	28%
episodic	27%
Improving: well in last 2½ years	11%
Acute: symptoms limited to first year	34%

3. SOCIAL OUTCOME

At 5 years (Wing)
In hospital during whole of 5-year period	11%
Severely disturbed in last 6 months	17%
Minor symptoms only: not working	16%
working	7%
Well and self-supporting	49%

Enormous improvement in proportion requiring long
term hospitalisation in recent decades (60% → 11%), but not much
change in proportion which show symptoms.

4. SOCIAL CORRELATES

Prevalence more common in social class V (likely to be due to
social drift because social class of fathers no different from
expectation).
Prognosis worse in social class V.

Social handicaps
   Primary: Due to florid symptoms.
   Secondary: Changed attitudes of others, loss of social contacts, impaired drive, general indifference (all worse with prolonged stay in hospital).
   Other: Poverty, lack of education, deprived of family support.

5. THE 'NEW LONG STAY' HOSPITAL PATIENTS (Mann & Cree)

In 1971, 21% of mental hospital patients had been there 1–5 years, of these 44.4% were schizophrenic.

6. AETIOLOGICAL THEORIES

Family environment
(Bateson) Parent-child relationship. Double bind communications involving incompatible opposites. Forced to decide between alternatives both of which are disapproved. Child forced into inactivity or ambiguous response.
   (Lidz) Whole family pathology. Close relationship with parent of opposite sex. Family dominated by the relationship. Other parent withdrawn, inadequate (skew). Hostile relationship in family (schism).
   (Wynne and Sanger) Family communication resembles schizophrenic psychopathology: fragmented, undirected. Possible to differentiate families of schizophrenic patients from normals in double blind control situation.
   (Laing) Schizophrenogenic mother: close, engulfing, exclusive, overprotective, ambivalent. Prevents maturation in child which doubts own feelings and sense of identity.
   Other family processes: blurred generation lines, psychological abnormalities of various kinds in first degree relatives, increased incidence of parental loss before 10 years.

Biochemical
Defect of amines and aminergic transmission. Functional excess or deficiency of amines involved in CNS transmission, or production of abnormal metabolites: due to error in metabolic pathway or variation in receptor sensitivity. Critique: uncertain whether toxic metabolites cause symptoms specifically analogous to those of schizophrenia. Difficult to control for metabolic changes caused by chronic hospitalisation.
   Indoleamine metabolism. Reduction of available serotonin may be basis for reserpine induced improvement in schizophrenia.
   Bad LSD 'trip' may resemble schizophrenia. Note that LSD affects serotonin-containing neurones and antagonises serotonin in vitro.

Epinephrine

Dopamine

5 Hydroxytryptamine
(Serotonin)

Mescaline

Methylated indoles can be psychotomimetic. There may be increased excretion of methylated indoles during relapse of schizophrenia.

Catecholamine metabolism. Epinephrine normally synthesised from phenylalanine via dopamine. Possible error of phenylalanine or epinephrine metabolism (oxidation, methylation). May be error of dopaminergic transmission.

Methylated catecholamines can be psychotomimetic. The hallucinogen mescaline (dimethoxyphenylethylamine) might be derived from dopamine.

Strong case that antipsychotic effects of neuroleptic drugs are due to block of dopamine receptors. Also evidence of abnormality of dopaminergic transmission in some schizophrenic patients.

Crow points out that dopamine hypothesis is of restricted application: neuroleptic drugs are of limited value in many chronic patients, who are also often resistant to the exacerbating effects of dexamphetamine which increases dopamine release. Suggests two distinct schizophrenic syndromes reflecting different pathological process: one characterised by 'positive' and the other by 'negative' symptoms.

	Syndrome I	Syndrome II
Symptoms	Positive (delusions, hallucinations, thought disorder)	Negative (affective flattening, poverty of speech, loss of volition)
Most common	in acute schizophrenia	in chronic schizophrenia

	Syndrome I	Syndrome II
Potential response to neuroleptic drugs	good	poor
Intellectual impairment	absent	sometimes present (correlates with increased ventricular size on CAT scan)
Outcome	reversible	? irreversible
Pathological process	increased dopamine receptors (post mortem evidence)	cell loss and structural brain changes, possibly encephalitic process

Mackay suggests that Syndromes I and II are both based on instability in control of dopaminergic transmission. Type I: overactivity, Type II: underactivity.

Genetic
1. Frequency of schizophrenia greater in families of patients than in controls. Life expectancy gen. pop'n. 0.9%, parents 5%, sibs. 8%, children 12%; DZ twins, opp. sex 6%, same sex 12%; MZ twins 58% (no significant difference reared together or separately).
2. Adult schizophrenics born of hospitalised schizophrenic mothers adopted at birth: 16.6% developed schizophrenia compared with none in controls (Heston U.S.A.).
3. Extended family study: excess of schizophrenic spectrum disorders in biological relatives of adopted adults who become schizophrenic (Kety, Denmark).
4. Adoptees with schizophrenic parent showed schizophrenic spectrum disorders twice as often as did controls (Rosenthal, Denmark).
5. Adoptive parent study: biological parents showed more psychological disturbance than adoptive parents of schizophrenics (Wender, U.S.A.).

Possible genetic mechanisms. Schizophrenics probably genetically heterogenous. Genetic predisposition interacts with environmental trigger. Polygenic theory is currently most popular (Gottesman and Shields). This accounts for threshold effects, gradation of severity, importance of non-genetic aetiological factors.

Environmental
Sharp increase in number of life events, some independent of patient's behaviour during three weeks prior to onset of acute illness. Most kinds of life events may trigger onset or relapse, often associated with stopping phenothiazine medication. Relapse less likely in situations of low emotional involvement and with work appropriate to capacity.

7. TREATMENT

Physical

Drugs

Phenothiazines. (Leff 1972) If maintained for one year after remission, 33% relapse compared with 83% controls. (Double blind design study of acute schizophrenia.)
   I.m. long acting preparations over nine month period: 8% relapsed compared with 66% placebo controls (may be effective when oral medication poorly absorbed: may precipitate severe depression in predisposed individuals: tardive dyskinesia). Avoidance of maintenance therapy may be justified if first illness with good prognostic signs. Otherwise continue 1–2 years after symptoms subside. Trial withdrawal should be gradual.

Thioxanthines. I.m. flupenthixol decanoate may be less likely to cause depression.

ECT
Not superior to drug therapy, but together with them may possibly lead to more rapid improvement.

Social
Manipulation of social forces with intention of reducing symptoms. Relapse more likely when return to situations with high emotional expressiveness and closeness.
   In chronic illness. Social stimulation leads to improvement while it occurs, but if excessive can cause relapse. Need adequate range of domestic environment with varying degrees of independence. Large custodial institutions can have adverse effects.

Psychological
Supportive attitudes in therapist, refuse to alienate or stereotype the patient, never patronise, look for meanings in psychotic symptoms, see regularly, listen, aim at recovery and assume this likely, allow maximal self-sufficiency compatible with clinical state. Interpretive therapy practised by some.

FURTHER READING

CLINICAL FEATURES

Granville-Grossman, K. (1971) *Recent Advances in Clinical Psychiatry-1*.
  Edinburgh: Churchill.
Mellor, C. S. (1982) The present status of first rank symptoms. *Brit. J.
  Psychiat.*, **140**, 423–424.

CAUSES

Biochemical

Frohman, C. E. & Gottlieb, J. S. (1974) In *American Handbook of Psychiatry*,
  2nd Edn, Vol. III, p. 601.
Mackay, A. V. P. & Crow, T. J. (1980) Positive and negative schizophrenic
  symptoms and the role of dopamine. *Brit. J. Psychiat.*, **137**, 379–387.

Genetic

Rosenthal, D. (1974). In *American Handbook of Psychiatry*, 2nd Edn, Vol. III,
  p. 588.

Interactional

Brown, G. W. (1967) The family of the schizophrenic patient. In *Recent
  Developments in Schizophrenia*. Kent: R.M.P.A. Headley.
Hirsch, S. R. & Leff, J. P. (1975) *Abnormalities in the Parents of
  Schizophrenics*: Maudsley monograph No. 22. London: Oxford University
  Press.

TREATMENT

Social

Wing, J. K. (1967) Social treatment, rehabilitation and management. In
  Recent Developments in Schizophrenia. Kent: R.M.P.A. Headley.

Drugs

Lipsedge, M. (1976) Drug treatment. In *Recent Advances in Clinical
  Psychiatry–2*. Ed. Granville-Grossman, K. Edinburgh: Churchill
  Livingstone.
Leff, J. P. (1972). Maintenance therapy and schizophrenia. *Brit. J. Hosp.
  Med.*, October.

Psychotherapy

Arieti, S. (1974). In *American Handbook of Psychiatry*, 2nd Edn, Vol. III,
  p. 627.
A useful series of articles on epidemiology, diagnosis and treatment in:
Brit. J. Hosp. Med., October 1972.

B. PARANOID STATES

NORMAL VARIANTS

Transient ideas of self reference may occur in normal, especially in sensitive, shy personalities.

Usually evanescent, carry no conviction and do not lead to action.

MORBID REACTIONS

More persistent with a sense of conviction, logic and coherence. May lead to action. Usually understandable in the light of situation and previous personality.

Causes
  1. *Acute organic brain syndromes* (drug or alcohol withdrawal delirium, post head injury, post operative, myxoedema). There may be marked paranoid ideas and acutely disturbed behaviour in context of confusion, disorientation and hallucinations.
  2. *Drug induced.* Amphetamine psychosis may closely resemble paranoid schizophrenia. LSD confusional hallucinatory states may contain paranoid element.
  3. Personality development. Certain self-referring individuals may develop systems of over-valued ideas, litiginous or otherwise in absence of other symptoms which might suggest psychosis. Morbid jealousy may be a highly dangerous state with intense jealous preoccupation regarding spouse, usually concerning infidelity. Often associated with impotence in male and previous alcohol abuse.
  4. *Situational.* Prolonged isolation, imprisonment, immigrant status.
     Folie à deux (Lasegue & Falret 1877) occurs in response to prolonged, more or less exclusive exposure to psychotic relative or other key individual, usually a dominant partner. Apparent delusional ideas may be identical in content with those of the psychotic individual, but more amenable to discussion and improve with separation.
     Folie simultanée occurs when the individuals are both psychotically ill.
     Group imitative disorders, especially under stress or in isolation (*folie à famille*).
  5. *Physical disability.* Deafness, especially in older persons. Less common in blindness. Disfiguring lesions, especially facial, deformed limbs and when acute in onset.
  6. *Complicating mental illness.* Paranoid symptoms especially common in the elderly. May complicate dementia of any kind

or affective disorders, but the cardinal symptoms of these remain discernible. Late onset paranoid schizophrenia similar and may present diagnostic difficulties.

C. AFFECTIVE DISORDERS

A group of illnesses of variable severity in which the central symptom is a periodic alteration of mood into either mania or depression, usually accompanied by other characteristic symptoms (Shaw).

EPIDEMIOLOGY

Female: male = 1.2–2.0/1.0
Prevalence of affective psychosis in general practice is 2.4–6.0/1000. This is ten times more than referral rate to hospital.
Lifetime morbidity rates in males = 4–18/1000 live births.
Lifetime morbidity rates in females = 6–28/1000 live births.

Natural history of illness
Recurrent relapses but without deterioration of personality between episodes. 40% readmitted at least once in four years after discharge from hospital (20% more than once).
  4–5% remain in hospital for one year compared with 14.5% patients suffering from schizophrenia (Norris 1955).
  Episodes become more frequent and their length tends to increase with age. May be recurrent depression or mania, or any sequence of the two. Circular (bipolar) forms with alternating mania and depression is uncommon and tends to follow a more malignant course.

SYMPTOMS AND SIGNS: DEPRESSIVE PSYCHOSIS

Overt depression of mood
May be diurnal variation, worse in morning.
Vary from flatness to deep gloom.
Tearfulness (particularly significant if different from previous personality).

Disorder of thinking
Pessimism. May see no future.
Suicidal ideas.
Poor concentration, mental slowness.
Delusional ideas: self-blame
                   nihilism
                   hypochondriacal
                   paranoid.
Impatience, irritability.

Motor concomitants
Poor appetite, weight loss.
Insomnia, especially early morning waking.
Retardation, stupor.
Agitation when anxiety marked.
Multiple somatic complaints.
Constipation.
Loss of libido.

Hallucinations
Usually auditory: critical voices.

Misinterpretations
Ideas of reference, e.g. people talking about self in a critical way.
Misconstrues remarks of others.

SYMPTOMS AND SIGNS: MANIC OR HYPOMANIC PSYCHOSIS

Elevation of mood
Persistent over days or weeks.
May be punctuated by episodic depression or irritability and angry
outbursts especially when wishes are thwarted.

Disorder of thinking
Flight of ideas: impaired train of thought related to pressure of
ideas and marked distractibility, impaired concentration.
Speech may contain puns, clang associations and rhyming in
context of euphoric mood.
Delusional ideas: re financial status, personal attributes. In a
minority may be paranoid.

Motor concomitants
Self-neglect, weight loss and exhaustion in severe cases.
Marked restlessness and overactivity.
Insomnia may be severe.
50% experience moderate/severe depression in first three months
of convalescence.
Mania may be confused with schizophrenic excitement.

CAUSAL THEORIES

Biochemical
May be more than one underlying chemical disorder.

Biogenic amine hypothesis
Clinical depression associated with a functional deficiency of nor
epinephrine or serotonin at receptor sites in brain. Mania
associated with excess of these agents.

Catecholamines. MAOIs increase intraneural concentration of active amines such as nor epinephrine, dopamine and serotonin. May also decrease their uptake. (Remains to be shown that MAOIs cause increased functional activity at central aminergic receptor sites).

Tricyclic antidepressants potentiate action of endogenously released nor epinephrine by blocking its reuptake into nerve terminals.

Reserpine causes depressive-like states and depletion of catecholamines.

Indoleamines. Antidepressants have similar effects on serotonin metabolism.

Some reports suggest that CSF 5 OH indoleacetic acid (breakdown product of serotonin) low in depression.

Increased hepatic tryptophan pyrrolase may reduce amount of tryptophan available for serotonin synthesis.

Tryptophan potentiates the antidepressant effect of MAOIs.

Fall in levels of 5HT may occur in parallel with changes in catecholamines.

Dewhurst Marley theory. Excitant (type A fat soluble) and Depressant (type C water soluble) amines with specific receptors. Depression due to deficiency in type A (e.g. tryptamine) or malfunction in type A receptor.

Change in receptor sensitivity (Ashcroft). Balance between transmitter availability and receptor sensitivity crucial.

Endocrine

Thyroid hormones may potentiate tricyclic antidepressants by influence on receptor sensitivity (activates adenyl cyclase-cyclic AMP system which is closely related to the adrenergic receptor).

Plasma adrenocortical steroids may be raised in severe depression. ? Related to nonspecific stress of the illness or disordered hypothalmic function.

Some claim that the limbic system and hypothalamus are the site of the primary pathology in the affective disorders. The dexamethasone suppression test has been used to evaluate the role of the hypothalamus-pituitary-adrenal cortex system (HPA). In normals there is suppression of plasma cortisol for 24 hours after overnight dose of dexamethasone. Depressed individuals show impaired suppression of plasma cortisol. Some authors claim that such findings are specific to 'endogenous' depression, especially when suicidal behaviour is present. The findings return to normal with recovery.

The suppression test may prove useful in diagnosis (e.g. distinguishing between organic dementia and pseudodementia in the elderly) and monitoring treatment.

Electrolyte metabolism
Electrolytes influence resting cell membrane potentials, impulse transmission and synaptic changes. Also have important role in biogenic amine release, reuptake and storage.

Lithium useful in therapy of affective disorders.

Intracellular sodium retention in depression, re-excretion in recovery (Gibbons).

Sodium retention may occur in Lithium responders.

Genetic

Familial incidence: MZ twins 74% concordance. DZ twins reared apart or together 19%. First degree relatives: 20% (manic depressive), 13% (uniphasic). General population 1%.

Unipolar and bipolar forms tend to breed true.

Possible genetic mechanisms. Single dominant autosomal gene. Incomplete penetrance because not all patients have affected parent, not all MZ twins concordant, rate less than 50% in sibs and children of patients.

Polygenic. This might explain continuum of severity of affective illnesses in general population.

Some degree of X-linkage. Greater than chance association with X linked marker traits, e.g. Xg blood system, dentan and protan colour blindness.

Psychological

Psychoanalytic. Loss of love object. Libido withdrawn and invested in the Ego which becomes identified with the lost object and subjected to sadistic impulses of the original ambivalent libidinous cathexis.

Early loss: severe depression associated with loss of parent before age of 20.

Severely depressed patients also show increased incidence of loss of parent through death during the 20 years preceding admission – applies only to patients under 40 years (Birtchnell).

Adaptation model. Depressive symptoms serve a protective purpose by reducing responsiveness (due to habituation through chronic frustration and lack of reinforcement).

Cognitive theory of depression. This postulates depressive syndrome as a process of 'cognitive shift' involving three areas of cognitive dysfunction.
These are:
Negative cognitive triad involving pervading themes related to the self, the world and the future.
Logical system errors leading to erroneous conclusions and

attitudes (arbitrary inference, selective abstraction, personalisation, overgeneralisation, magnification, minimisation).
Idiosyncratic schemes which act as enduring cognitive templates which screen, code, categorise and evaluate information.

'Reactive' v 'endogenous' depression

Neurotic (reactive)	Psychotic (endogenous)
Reactivity of depression	Disturbance of food intake, weight
Rapid mood changes	Delusions:
Psychological precipitation	guilt
Hysterical + anxiety symptoms	unworthiness
Previous symptoms:	bodily change
hysterical	persecution
anxiety	Ideas of reference
obsessional	Suspiciousness
bodily preoccupation	Perplexity
mood variation	Severe insomnia
Childhood neurotic traits	Apathy
Irritability	Agitation
Hypochondriacal attitude	Social withdrawal
Demonstrative suicidal attempt	Speech: abnormal rate or quantity
Suicidal feelings	Auditory hallucinations
Poor response to	Family history of affective
antidepressants, ECT	psychosis
	Good response to
	antidepressants, ECT

Bimodal distribution of symptoms (Newcastle) suggests two distinct clinical entities. Kendell suggests this finding might be an artefact due to patient selection and 'halo' effects: when consecutive patients rated, distribution is unimodal. The two syndromes may be at opposite ends of depressive continuum, most patients fall somewhere between, having a mixture of both kinds of symptom.

Linear relation between score on neurotic/psychotic scale and response to ECT. Multiple causation compatible with this.

Social: the Brown and Harris Study

Depressed women in urban community. Interviewed 114 psychiatric patients and 458 women in random community sample. Assessed situational and life-event causal factors: emphasis placed not merely on change but also its meaning for the individual. Formulated causal theory of depression which accords central importance to social factors. Life events relevant only if perceived as long-term threat.

Provoking factors
Either severe event or major life difficulty. 'Severe event' defined as experience of loss or disappointment concerning a person, object, role or idea (e.g. real or threatened separation from key figure, major material loss, general disappointment, miscellaneous crises such as work redundancy). 'Major life difficulties' were those of at least 2 years duration (excluding problems of health).

15% of women were considered to have suffered from affective disorder in the 3 months before interview. 8% were 'onset cases' in which depression had commenced at some time in the previous year.

83% of onset cases had experienced severe event or major life difficulty.

61% of cases   } had experienced at least one severe
19% of non cases } event in the preceding nine months
29% of patients did not have provoking factors

Provoking factors important in both psychotic and neurotic depression. Only 20% of provoking factors followed by depression, the development of which requires the presence of vulnerability factors.

Vulnerability factors
These become causal only in the presence of provoking agent. They do not in themselves lead to depression.
They are: — absence of intimate relationship
           — lack of mother (not father) before age 11 years
           — lack of employment outside home
They act by lowering self esteem, thereby impairing ability to cope with provoking factors and leading to the central depressive triad in which the self seems worthless, the future hopeless and the world meaningless. They are more common in working-class women, and explain why these are four times more likely than middle-class women to develop depressive disorder in face of provoking agent. The class difference is restricted to women with children. Less important cause of social class difference was increased experience of severe life events and major life difficulties in working-class women.

Symptom formation factors
These are related to the overall severity of depression.
They are — past loss
       — age over 40 years
       — previous episode
The presence of all three symptom formation factors strongly related to absence of provoking agent.

Psychotic depression related to loss by death
Neurotic depression related to loss by separation

INVOLUTIONAL MELANCHOLIA

Not a distinct entity: depression in elderly does not differ in any fundamental way from that in younger patients either symptomatically or genetically. Hypochondriacal delusions probably due to pathoplastic effects of age.

TREATMENT OF DEPRESSIVE ILLNESS

Psychotherapy
Supportive relationship can be very beneficial. See regularly. Avoid facile reassurance although maintain an optimistic approach. Investigate physical symptoms only on their intrinsic merit, not merely to reassure. Dissuade from major changes in life, e.g. resignation from job when depressed or hypomanic. Hospital admission if: persistent disabling affective symptoms, significant risk of suicide, poor social support or family intolerance hinder recovery. Use interpretive psychotherapy after affective symptoms resolved: aim to clarify precipitating factors and facilitate adjustment to them, involve 'key other' persons in therapy where possible. Early causal factors may also be discussed in more prolonged formal therapy.

Cognitive therapy
An active directive time-limited structured approach. May be used in a variety of disorders. In the treatment of depression it aims to help the patient to
— develop a more positive attitude
— stop unjustified thoughts which negate this view
— adopt thoughts that uphold it.
  Appeal to facts of day to day behaviour (use of diary) in order to disprove false ideas.
  Useful in mild to moderate depression, particularly as adjunct to physical methods of treatment, or alone when these are inappropriate.

Drugs

Pharmacology of antidepressant drugs

Tricyclics: tertiary amines (e.g. amitriptyline, imipramine, clomipramine, trimipramine, doxepin, dibenzepin). Other drugs such as chlorpromazine may compete with enzymic oxidation in liver, with resulting slower breakdown.
  Adjustment of dose relatively easy because response increases with dose which can be pushed to limit of tolerance.

Tricyclics: secondary amines (e.g. nor-triptyline, desimipramine, protriptyline): effectiveness may be reduced in high doses.

All tricyclic antidepressants reduce the uptake of hypertensive agents into adrenergic neurones and renders them ineffective. Avoid combining the two. Their atropine-like action may cause serious synergism with other drugs and lead to glaucoma, ileus, urinary retention.

Overdose may cause coma, convulsions, hypertension, cardiac dysrhythmias, and hallucinations during recovery.

Mono amine oxidase inhibitors (MAOIs): mono amine oxidase enzymes block intestinal absorption of tyramine which is an indirect sympathomimetic amine: does not act on adrenergic receptors but provokes release of catecholamines which cause hypertension with or without hyperpyrexia.

MAOIs block the intestinal protective mechanism, and foods containing sufficient tyramine may cause dangerous reactions.

Foods to be avoided: mature cheeses, pickled herrings, yeast, meat extracts (Marmite, Bovril), Chianti, beer, sherry, game, badly stored meat, any protein food that is not fresh, banana skins, broad bean pods (dopa).

MAOIs interact with:
a. Tyramine-like drugs, which include amphetamine, mephentermine and other pressors, ephedrine, phenylephrine and other nasal decongestants, phenylpropanolamine (proprietary cough and cold cures), fenfluramine, phenmetrazine, chlorphentermine, and other amphetamine-like anti-obesity agents, levodopa.
b. Tricyclic antidepressants, especially when MAOIs have been commenced first. Must be free from MAOIs *as well as* tricyclic drugs for 1 week before starting combined therapy. If one is discontinued, it may not be safe to restart. Use of combined therapy is best left to specialist centres.
c. Other MAOIs. Always leave an interval of time before changing from one to another.
d. Miscellaneous. Pethidine, α methyl dopa, reserpine, may potentiate hypoglycaemic drugs, prolong action of barbiturates, chloral hydrate and alcohol.

Metabolism of MAOIs: in 46% rapid acetylation occurs with poor response. Need flexible dosage programme.

Tryptophane may potentiate antidepressant effect of MAOIs.

Mortality of therapy with antidepressant drugs: annual deaths (per 10^6 prescription): amitriptyline 2.3, phenelzine 17.2.

Tricyclics may predispose to sudden death under stress, the risk increased $\times$ 8 with exercise in cold. Cardiac dysrhythmias may complicate overdose.

N.B. 15% of individuals with affective psychosis eventually die through suicide.

Drug management of depression
(See Shaw)

Tricyclic initially, sufficient tertiary amine type drug to cause mild side effects for 4 weeks, then 7–10 days at slightly lower dose. First choice when patient mildly or moderately ill in absence of heart disease (amitriptyline 75 mg, single dose at night, increasing to 150 mg after 4 days). If ineffective in 28 days, no point in continuing.

If using secondary amine type drug and no response, reduce dose slightly in case optimal dose is low.

Newer antidepressants. Flupenthixol: low toxicity. Useful in elderly; depot decanoate available.

Tetracyclics: (Mianserin, maprotiline).

MAOIs. Not all clinicians accept their use as justifiable. Patients should be able to exercise dietary discretion and avoid impulsive overdoses. Contraindicated when arteriosclerosis or liver disease present.

Phenelzine: dose difficult to judge because of variable rate of acetylation.

Isocarboxazid: weak but useful in older patients, 20–30 mg per day.

Tranylcypromine: more reliable. Stimulant. 20 mg mane, 10 mg midday, for 3 weeks. Usually effective with 3 weeks' treatment at doses causing mild side effects such as postural hypotension. Maximum dose 60 mg daily.

ECT in depression
First choice therapy in moderate/severe depression when suicidal risk serious and/or little response to drug therapy. May need 3–4 unilateral treatments in first week if severe. Maximum of 12 applications in one course.

TREATMENT OF MANIA

(See Shaw)

Psychotherapy
As in depression.

Drugs
Haloperidol: drug of first choice. 10–30 mg i.m. Monitor blood pressure — should not fall below 100 mgHg systolic. Repeat at 1–1½ hr intervals until mania subsides: may need 40–100 mg per day initially. Switch to oral therapy as soon as possible (oral dose = 2 × i.m. dose).

Lithium carbonate: commence at same time as haloperidol, delay of 10 days before it acts. 0.8–1.0 mEq/L. Dose 1000–1200 mg per day. Check serum level every 5 days initially.

Phenothiazines: if chlorpromazine used, give test dose 10 mg i.m. and monitor for hypotension. 50–75 mg i.m. every 30–45 minutes until improvement occurs. Only give antiparkinsonian drugs if needed.

TREATMENT OF RECURRENT AFFECTIVE ILLNESS

Tricyclic antidepressants maintained for 6 months after episode of depression reduces risk of relapse. Not effective in mania or bipolar illnesses.

If maintenance lithium proposed: check renal, cardiac functions and make sure not pregnant or planning to be. Stop lithium if become pregnant.

Check blood levels if intercurrent disease or currently taking diuretics (exactly 12 hours after last dose).

Side effects of lithium: nausea, loose stools, vomiting, diarrhoea, tremor of hands (coarse tremor may herald serious toxicity), polyuria, polydipsia, weight gain, oedema, sluggishness, sleepiness, vertigo, dysarthria. Occasionally hypo thyroid goitre (treat with 0.1–0.2 mg thyroxin daily, but may have to stop lithium). May be fatal coma in severe overdosage. Slow excretion of drug makes treatment of overdose difficult.

FURTHER READING

Ashcroft, G. W. (1974) Biogenic amines. *Medicine*, 1757–1761.
Beck, A. T. (1976) Cognitive therapy and the emotional disorders. New York: International Universities Press.
Beck, A.T. Rush, B. F., & Emery, G. (1979) Cognitive therapy of depression. New York: Guildford Press.
Birtchnell, J. (1970) Depression in relation to early and recent parental death. *Brit. J. Psychiat.*, **116**, 229–306.
Brown, G. W. et al. (1977) Depression and loss. *Brit. J. Psychiat.*, **130**, 1–18.
Brown, G. W., & Harris, T. (1978) Social origins of depression. London: Tavistock.
Granville-Grossman, K. L. (1968). The early environment in affective disorders. In: *Recent Developments in Affective Disorders*, Ed. Coppen & Walk. Ashford: Headley Bros.
Carroll, B. J. (1982). The dexamethasone suppression test for melancholia. *Brit. J. Psychiat.*, **140**, 292–304.
Kendell, R. E. (1968) *The Classification of Depressive Illness*.
Maudsley Monograph No. 18. London: Oxford University Press.
Mendels, J. (1974) Biological aspects of affective illness. In *American Handbook of Psychiatry*. Ed. S. Arieti, 2nd Edn. Vol. III, p. 491–523.
Rawnsley, K. (1968) Epidemiology of affective disorders. In *Recent Developments in Affective Disorders*. Ed. Coppen and Walk. Ashford: Headley Bros.

Shaw, D. M. (1973) Biochemical basis of affective disorders. *Brit. J. Hosp. Med.*, Nov. 1973, 609–616.

Shaw, D. M. (1977) The practical management of affective disorders. *Brit. J. Psychiat.*, **130**, 430–451.

BEREAVEMENT REACTIONS

Typical (uncomplicated) grief
Initial short period of emotional 'numbness'.

Episodic emotional distress, becoming less severe in 1–2 months.

Off work for short periods (2 weeks). No psychiatric consultation needed.

Severity and type of distress may vary even within the same individual from one episode of bereavement to another, depending on the precise nature of the loss in each instance. Disturbing sense of loss may last many months.

Preoccupation with memories of the deceased
May be clear visual imagery.
Idealise the dead person.

Perceptual disturbances
Misinterpret sounds as due to the deceased.
Misidentify other persons as being the deceased.
Sense of presence.
Visual hallucinations, occasional auditory.

Mental distress
Depression, withdrawal, guilt (suicidal ideas 11%).
Episodic yearning, anxiety.

Physical symptoms
Headaches, vomiting, anorexia, chest pains, dyspnoea, joint pains (may resemble those in dead person's final illness).

Behavioural changes
Social withdrawal, restlessness. Conduct aimed at keeping memory alive.
Preservation of possessions (mummification).

Hostility
Anger at those responsible for care of the deceased during terminal illness.
Loss of compassion for others.
Anger at being abandoned.

Increased mortality risk
4.76% first degree relatives in first year, 0.86% controls. (Rees &
Lutkins.)
Suicide increased × 2.5 in first year. Risk greatest in widowers. 40%
increase in death from coronary thrombosis, cancer, respiratory
infections.

Long term effects
Childhood bereavement may predispose to psychiatric illness in
adulthood, particularly depression. Increased risk of alcoholism in
men. Chronic poor physical health (43%).

Atypical (complicated) grief

May take various forms
Absence of grief.
Excessively delayed (related to phobic avoidance, extreme guilt,
anger).
Unduly prolonged (often anger over care of deceased).
More severe (suicide attempts, excessive guilt, severe depression,
anger, intense social withdrawal).
Psychosomatic symptoms may predominate (e.g. hypertension,
diabetes, duodenal ulcer, asthma, ulcerative colitis).
Certain symptoms particularly common: difficulty in accepting the
loss (refusal), marked hostility to others, identification with
personality traits and symptoms of deceased, excessive
idealisation, recurrent nightmares, avoidance of memories, objects
or places associated with deceased, anniversary reactions, panic
attacks.

More common when bereaved person:
Has had previous psychiatric difficulties.
Was excessively dependent on deceased.
Had ambivalent or otherwise difficult relationship with deceased.

Treatment
Helping the work of grieving: realisation, making real the loss,
disengagement. Formal ritual aspects of mourning help.

Helping strategies
Listen, encourage to express feelings (especially after the funeral is
over). Psychotropic drugs when symptoms severe. Self-help
groups (beware they do not encourage perpetuation of grief).
Exploit social 'bridges' at turning point in grief.
   Morbid grief may be resistant to treatment. When *avoidance
behaviour* predominates, a 'forced mourning' procedure is often
effective (Lieberman).

Forced mourning ineffective, perhaps harmful, in those who have inadequate family support and significant social problems.

Other relatives may share morbid grief and may also be included in forced mourning procedure.

FURTHER READING

Brown, G. W. et al. (1977) Depression and loss. *Brit. J. Psychiat.*, **130**, 1–18.

Granville-Grossman, K. (1971) In: *Recent Advances in Clinical Psychiatry – 1*, pp. 180–191. Edinburgh: Churchill Livingstone.

Lieberman, S. (1978) Nineteen cases of morbid grief. *Brit. J. Psychiat.*, **132**, 159–163.

Parkes, C. M. (1972) *Bereavement: Studies of Grief in Adult Life*. London: Tavistock.

Rees, W. D. & Lutkins, S. G. (1967) Mortality of bereavement. *Brit. Med. J.*, **4**, 13–16.

The neuroses

A. HYSTERIA

A psychological reaction usually at an unconscious level and related to chronic unresolved internal conflict or acute external stress.

May show belle indifference: lack of anxiety and concern over disability caused by hysterical symptoms.

CLINICAL FEATURES

Symptoms of two types

a. Conversion
Psychogenic disorder of bodily function greater than normal psychosomatic interaction. May take form of paralysis, ataxia, tremor, blindness, deafness, pseudo epilepsy, syncope. Pain may be the most common. May include a variety of psychological symptoms e.g. hallucinations, depression.

Conversion symptoms can be distinguished from those due to organic disease by:
1. variability
2. lack of objective evidence of organic disease
3. atypicality (e.g. disturbance of sensory loss, type of ataxia)
4. inconsistency (apparently paralysed muscles may show normal power when acting as synergists, or weakness may be due to contraction of antagonists)
5. loss of function reflects patient's concept of disability rather than neuro anatomical principles.

b. Dissociation
Psychogenic disorders involving impairment of personal awareness. May take the form of amnesia, clouding, apparent disorientation, with or without fugue state, alternate personality.

Dissociative amnesia often global, involving total recall in absence of evidence of organic brain disorder but with retention of registration, of evidence of organic brain disorder but with retention of registration, recall for immediate past, and skills in reading, writing and arithmetic. May selectively involve memory loss for emotionally upsetting events.

Secondary gain
This is frequently discernible.

May complicate true organic disease
This may present with symptoms which are partly or completely due to hysterical mechanisms.

Temporal lobe epilepsy particularly liable to precipitate hysterical symptoms.

Of 85 patients with 'hysteria' followed up 9 years later, 66% were found to have developed florid organic disease: this had not been detected clinically when hysteria diagnosed at first, but had probably played a part in leading to initial symptoms (Slater).

Symptom groupings (Reed)
113 patients: detailed clinical analysis and follow up mean 11.7 years.
A. 13% conversion/dissociative only. No other symptoms developed. Often single illness.
B. 33% conversion/dissociative with affective symptoms (depression, anxiety, preceded or followed original episode).
C. 28% affective symptoms only. More aptly termed histrionic behaviour.
D. 21% other syndromes present (e.g. schizophrenia, agoraphobia).
E. 5% uncertain diagnosis.

Concludes: Group A represents discrete syndrome of pure 'hysteria' characterised by conversion/dissociation, belle indifference and secondary gain in absence of other symptoms.

Clinical syndromes (Merskey)
A. Single motor, sensory or dissociative symptoms, sometimes including pain.
B. Polysymptomatic e.g. hypochondriasis and *Briquet's* syndrome.
C. Elaboration of organic complaint.
D. Self induced illness or self damage in abnormal personality.
E. Psychotic or pseudo psychotic disorders (Ganser Syndrome, hysterical/psychosis).
F. Culturally sanctioned: endemic or epidemic.

Munchausen syndrome
Recurrent presentation to hospitals, simulated organic disease, may lead to unnecessary major medical or surgical intervention. Some cases follow episodes of true organic disease. Seek relief in sick role. Level of conscious awareness of underlying motives uncertain. Formulation mainly in terms of malingering, inadequate.

AETIOLOGY

Slater suggests there is no such entity as hysteria, merely hysterical symptoms which may complicate other conditions.

Reed distinguishes a pure entity of 'hysteria' and provided it is strictly defined, argues for its retention.

Psychoanalytic theory

Repressed anxiety due to instinctual impulses lead to hysterical symptoms which often have symbolic meaning and secondary gain. Radical resolution of conflict is avoided. In some cases this may be sexual: the Oedipus complex (the nuclear process in the neurosis) is seen as particularly relevant to hysteria, remaining at the phallic phase of sexual development (Fenichel). Phobic anxiety seen as form of anxiety hysteria, repressed anxiety, displaced on to neutral object or situation.

Genetic

Increased incidence of hysteria in relatives of hysterics, but they also show a similar increase in variety of other conditions (Ljungberg). No significant twin concordance.

Suggestion and shared anxiety

Outbreaks of mass hysteria in certain communities. Charcot produced hysterical symptoms by strong suggestion and saw hysteria as disease entity.

Personality

In 40% of cases of hysteria, preceding 'hysterical' traits: dependent, manipulative, egocentric, attention seeking, histrionic, labile and superficial emotionality.

Beware of pejorative misuse of these terms. Chodoff urges that we discard the concept of hysterical personality: dubious validity and uncertain relationships to hysteria.

Patients with hysterical pain have characteristic high MMPI scores for hypochondriasis and hysteria, low for depression. (The V triad.)

Sick role

Seek this through learnt behaviour in face of intolerable life difficulties, conflict or physical disease. Variable degree of conscious awareness of mechanism for symptoms, and delineation from malingering often highly arbitrary.

Compensation neurosis

More common in less severe injuries and in those involving compensation. Improvement when claim is settled. May be related to poor verbal fluency, more common in social classes IV and V and in poorly educated, particularly recent immigrants.

TREATMENT

Rapid spontaneous recovery of acute reactions when removed from causative stress. Communication model often useful: concentrates on the meaning of the disability conveyed to others or in terms of internal conflict. Emphasise psychotherapy when reaction is based on long-standing emotional conflict. Avoid undue preoccupation with physical symptoms: investigate them only as far as medically indicated not merely as a method of reassurance. Minimise advantages of sick role.

PROGNOSIS

Depends on the associated condition, environmental problems and resilience of personality or causative problems.

Good: Acute onset, nature of conflict clear, resolvable social factors or related to drug intoxication.

Poor: Related to intractible personality or situational problems, patient remains hostile and unwilling to cooperate in treatment.

Ljungberg: 43% males, 35% females had residual symptoms after 1 year.

Lewis: 40% well and working 5 years later (Maudsley Hospital inpatients).

Carter: 70% well 4–6 years later (acute conversion reaction).

FURTHER READING

SYMPTOMS

Merskey, H. (1978) *Brit. J. Hosp. Med.*, **19**, 305–310.

DIAGNOSIS

Chodoff, P. (1974) *Am. J. Psychiat.*, **131**, 1073–1078.
Fenichel, O. (1945) *The Psychoanalytic Theory of Neurosis.* New York: Norton.
Kendell, R. E. *Medicine* (1972–1974 Series) 1780–1783.
Reed, J. L. (1975) *Psychological Medicine*, **5**, 13–17.
Reed, J. L. (1978) Compensation neurosis and Munchausen syndrome. *Brit. J. Hosp. Med.*, **19**, 314–325.
Slater, E. (1965) *Brit. Med. J.*, **1**, 1395–1399.

THE GANSER SYNDROME

The syndrome

Ganser 1897 described syndrome in 3 prisoners as an 'Unusual Hysterical Confusional State':

Disordered consciousness with subsequent amnesia.
Hallucinations.

Sensory changes of hysterical type.
Vorbiereden (approximate and absurd answers).
Abrupt termination.
Rare to see complete syndrome but Ganser-type symptoms more common (Scott, Whitlock).
Not necessarily restricted to prison populations.
Uncertain whether primarily hysterical, organic confusion or schizophrenic reaction.
Verbal responses resemble early stage of dysphasia.
Difficult to define concept of 'approximate' answers: may be more in nature of random responses (some correct, other absurd).
May complicate variety of other illnesses — organic brain disease or psychotic states. Clouding of consciousness essential, otherwise suspect hysterical pseudo dementia, malingering or buffoonery type schizophrenia.

FURTHER READING

Scott, P. D. (1965) *Brit. J. Criminology*, **5**, 127–134.
Whitlock, F. A. (1965) *Brit. J. Psychiat.*, **113**, 12–29.

B. OBSESSIONAL COMPULSIVE STATES

HISTORY

Janet emphasised irresolute hesitant attitudes (Folie du doute) and introduced concept of a single neurosis encompassing variety of phenomena. Coined term 'psychasthenia': a failure of will and attention, pathological diminution of mental energy.

Epidemiology
68% onset before 25 years of age. Average age onset 22.5 years (SD 12.1 years).
Morbid risk decreases with increasing age.
More common in females.

PHENOMENOLOGY

SYMPTOMS

Abnormal mental content (idea, image, impulse or movement) having a subjective sense of compulsion over-riding an internal resistance. Recognised by the patient on quiet reflection as being abnormal and irrational. Obsessional ideas (ruminations) are subjective mental events. Compulsive rituals abnormal and irrational, involve motor movement. Resistance is associated with increased anxiety. Repetition an important feature, associated only with transient anxiety reduction.
Distinguish from delusional ideas which may also be repetitive

and preoccupying, but are regarded by the patient as logical and true.

Affective symptoms such as phobias are only strictly obsessional if they possess all the diagnostic criteria, e.g. fear associated with obsessional compulsive symptoms.

Content often concerned with fear of harming, or contaminating others. Cleaning behaviour and avoidance of fearful stimuli the most common compulsive features. Primary ideas may lead to secondary rituals e.g. washing which then becomes obsessional in quality. Criminal obsessional acts rare but in small minority self control may be overwhelmed, especially when previous personality shows recurrent aggressive behaviour, alcohol abuse is present, or depression is marked. Obsessional fears of harming baby may develop in puerperium: need to distinguish from depressive psychosis where risk of harming self and/or baby is severe.

AETIOLOGY

Need to distinguish childhood ritualistic play behaviour which is common and normal.

Psychological theory
Defect in arousal system: major defensive reaction precipitated by minor stimuli. Leads to placatory activity which serves as a failure defence in the control of unpleasant internal states (Beech).

Anankastic personality
Carries increased risk: excessive preoccupation with orderliness, cleanliness, vacillating, conscientious, checking, anxiety prone, rigid.

Complicating other illness
Depressive illness (found in 20%): close relation with depression, both have periodic course.
Anorexia nervosa (20%)
Schizophrenia
Early Dementia
Post encephalitis lethargica (uncertain whether strictly obsessional/compulsive).

Psychoanalytic theory
Defensive regression to anal sadistic phase of development leading to ambivalence, magical thinking, fear of effects of obsessional thoughts, increase in number of taboo objects with punitive superego. Due to conflict at oedipal genital stage of libidinal development.

Defence mechanisms against unconscious aggressive impulses.

Secondary gain
May be an initiating or perpetuating factor.

TREATMENT

Ensure that depressive symptoms are effectively treated.

Drugs
Do not use electively but may be necessary to control severe affective disturbance. Anafranil useful.

Psychotherapy
Supportive type valuable. Insight-directed formal therapy difficult. Secondary gain may impede progress.
May need conjoint approach with spouse or 'key other'.

Behaviour therapy
Rituals. A significant proportion helped by response prevention. Admit to hospital, 24 hour monitoring, strong dissuasion, provision of alternative behaviour. Based on principle that repetition is a pathogenic factor in encouraging and consolidating rituals. Modelling involves the therapist touching feared objects, then encouraging patient to do so. Similar to flooding. Useful to carry out this approach in patient's home after discharge from inpatient care: involve family in modelling. Based on extinction process.

Obsessional thoughts. More difficult to treat, not amenable to behaviour therapy. Thought stopping involves encouraging to switch train of thought.

Leucotomy
Sometimes used as last resort when illness is severe and in danger of becoming chronic (2–3 years duration), good previous personality, no aggressive traits, physically well, absence of significant interpersonal or social causal factors. The 1983 Mental Health Act requires consent as well as a second medical and two non-medical opinions in all patients.

PROGNOSIS

Episodic course with remissions common. Basic amelioration rate: 66% fully well or much improved and leading normal life 5 years after onset. 79% illness episodes last less than 1 year (Pollitt).
Improvement may await changes in environmental perpetuating factors.
Rarely leads to development of psychotic illness: only slight increase in incidence of psychosis in relatives.

Poor outcome
Marked mood disorder (anxiety, depression, anger). Long duration of symptoms before treatment commenced. Reluctance to accept help.

FURTHER READING

Beech, H. R. (1978) Advances in the treatment of obsessional neurosis. *Brit. J. Hosp. Med.*, Jan. 54–60.
Crowe, M. J. (1976) Behavioural treatment in psychiatry. In *Recent Advances in Clinical Psychiatry–2.* Ed. K. Granville-Grossman. Edinburgh: Churchill Livingstone.
Dowson, J. H. (1977) The phenomenology of obsessional compulsive neurosis. *Brit. J. Psychiat.*, **131**, 75–79.
Grimshaw, L. (1965) The outcome of obsessional disorder: follow up of 100 cases. *Brit. J. Psychiat.*, **111**, 1051–1056.
Pollitt, J. D. (1957) Natural history of obsessional states: a study of 150 cases. *Brit. Med. J.*, **1**, 194–198.

C. PHOBIC ANXIETY

DEFINITION

A phobia is a special form of fear which is out of proportion to the demands of a situation, cannot be explained or reasoned away, is beyond voluntary control and leads to avoidance of the feared situation (Marks).

Usually many physical autonomic concomitants of anxiety.

CLINICAL TYPES

Related to external stimuli
Most common:
　　Agoraphobia 60%
　　Social Phobia 8%
　　Animal Phobia 3%
　　Miscellaneous specific phobias 14%

Related to internal stimuli
Illness phobia, hypochondriasis.
Obsessive phobias.

Agoraphobia
Commonest and most distressing. 66% are females. 6.3 per 1000 general population, onset 18–35 years of age. Fear of open spaces, often also for going out alone, into crowds, travelling, closed spaces.

Usually accompanied by diverse anxiety symptoms. Social anxiety common. Family often stable, closely knit.

History of childhood fears (night terrors), enuresis in 55%.

Sexual frigidity in 60% female patients (significantly more than control group). Less common in males: antedates or follows agoraphobic symptoms. Onset in some follows traumatic event with situational panic.

Avoidance of phobic situation may be marked, aimed at anxiety reduction.

Secondary involvement of family common.

Symptoms may serve secondary gain.

Associated non-phobic symptoms:
— general anxiety
— depersonalisation (37%)
— depression
— obsessional compulsive phenomena.

Specific animal phobias
Majority commence before puberty. Many remit as relearning occurs. Less likely to have multiple associated anxiety symptoms. Contrast agoraphobia.

Social phobias
May lead to gross restriction of activities because of self conscious fears. Onset usually after puberty.

Illness phobias
Hypochondriasis (multiple fears). Nosophobia (fear of specific illness). May be symptomatic of other condition:
— lasting personality trait e.g. obsessional.
— depressive or schizophrenic illness.
— response to anxiety or stress.
Previous health history or illness in relative may be relevant.

Obsessive phobias
Fear of contaminating or harming others or the self.
Repeatedly intrude into consciousness despite resistance.
No fear of the object, only the consequences therefrom.
Usually with compulsive washing, avoidance rituals.
Risk of acting-out fears is small in absence of significant depression or aggressive personality disorder.
Desensitisation difficult because extremely specific to each feared situation and little generalisation.

TREATMENT

Initial full assessment of the total situation essential.

1. Systematic desensitisation

Most effective in focal circumscribed phobias. Gradual exposure to phobic stimuli along hierarchy of increasing intensity. Practice in fantasy (imaginal) together with situational. Results superior to other methods. Benefits may accrue even in chronic agoraphobia. Problems may occur: achieving deep relaxation, providing vivid imagery of phobia, irrelevant/fluctuating hierarchy, lack of motivation due to life situational problems.

Facilitated by: muscular and mental relaxation, expectation, reassurance, practice and suggestion by therapist, practice of regime, discourage avoidance behaviour, positive involvement of relatives. Poor response in agoraphobia, severe obsessions, high overt (free floating) anxiety with marked physiological correlates of anxiety.

2. Modelling (vicarious learning)

Observing model (therapist, relative) engage in non-avoidance behaviour with the feared stimulus.

3. Flooding (implosion)

In vivo or imaginal. Encourage maximal supervised exposure to feared stimulus as rapidly as possible until anxiety reduction is experienced. Prolonged exposure may provide lasting improvement e.g. 4–5 hours over 2–3 days.

4. Paradoxical intention (logotherapy)

Seek out and encourage to expose self to phobic stimulus.

5. Relaxation techniques and hypnotic suggestion

6. Psychotherapy

Especially when other personality difficulties, secondary gain present. May need conjoint therapy with relative. Commitment and attitude of therapist important.

7. Drug therapy

Minor tranquillisers and antidepressants when relevant symptoms severe. Avoid prolonged courses. Use in anticipation of situational exposure.

NATURAL HISTORY, PROGNOSIS

Fluctuant course, tendency to relapse with panic attacks. If acute situational precipitant, tends to clear gradually unless reinforced by repeated trauma or when prolonged avoidance of feared situation has occurred. When persistent for more than 1 year spontaneous recovery unlikely. If secondary to depressive illness improvement occurs as this remits. Agoraphobia tends to improve slowly without treatment. Animal phobias do not. After desensitisation: agoraphobia 45% much improved in 1 year. Other phobias 55% much improved in 1 year. (Marks and Gelder.)

D. THE HYPERVENTILATION SYNDROME

The most common psychophysiological reaction due to anxiety encountered by physicians (Pincus). Focusses anxiety on organs by causing symptoms in them. Common in young females (29% of those aged 15–30 years referred for neurological opinion).

SYMPTOMS

Faintness, visual disturbance, poor concentration.
Nausea, vertigo.
Fullness in head, chest, epigastrium.
Headache.
Breathlessness, palpitation, hot flushes, cold sweats.
Paraesthesiae, vomiting.

CAUSE

Calibre of cerebral blood vessels closely related to p CO_2 in blood.
Four minutes overbreathing can reduce cerebral blood flow by 40%. Secondary alkalosis, tetany, fits.
May accentuate cerebral dysrhythmia in epileptics.
Exaggerated by orthostatic hypotension, valsalva manoeuvre.

DIAGNOSTIC TEST

Symptoms reproduced by 3 minutes overbreathing.

FURTHER READING

Boulougouris, J. C. & Marks I. M. (1969) Implosion (flooding). A new treatment for phobias. *Brit. Med. J.*, **2**, 721–723.
Lipsedge, M. S. (1973) Systematic desensitisation. *Brit. J. Hosp. Med.*, (May) 657–664.
Marks, I. M. (1969) *Fears and Phobias*. London: Heinemann Medical.
Pincus, J. H. (1978) Hyperventilation syndrome. *Brit, J. Hosp. Med.*, (April) **19**, 312–313.
Watson, J. P., Gaind, R. & Marks, I. M. (1971) Prolonged exposure: a rapid treatment of phobia. *Brit. Med. J.*, **1**, 13–15.

Personality disorders

These are enduring aspects of psychological make up in the individual. Unwise to make this diagnosis in adolescence when major potential for change still present.

Adequate evaluation of personality characteristics permit fuller evaluation of: the rate of development of any psychiatric illness, the extent of change from 'normal self', relevant precipitating factors, realistic treatment goals.

TYPES

Paranoid: either sensitive and blaming others or somewhat aggressive preoccupation with personal rights. Both have an excessive tendency to self reference, may also have 'over-valued' ideas.

Affective (cyclothymic): persistent anomalies of mood — depressive, euphoric or alternating between these.

Schizoid: extreme reserve, shyness, aloofness, may be eccentric behaviour.

Explosive: instability of mood, liable to sudden irritability, anger, impulsive aggression. At other times normal and not antisocial.

Anankastic (obsessive, compulsive): extremely cautious, conscientious, rigid, perfectionist, vacillating and doubting. Prone to anxiety, may show obsessional traits such as checking.

Hysterical: shallow, labile affective features, over-dependence on others. Erratic relationships, may be histrionic and may develop hysterical symptoms under stress.

Asthenic: passive dependent, lack of resilience and mental vigour.

Antisocial: persistent antisocial behaviour with lack of sympathetic feeling or remorse. May be abnormally aggressive. Includes psychopathic disorder as defined under the Mental Health Act 1983 as a persistent disorder or disability of mind (whether or not including significant impairment of intelligence) which results in abnormally aggressive or seriously irresponsible conduct on the part of the person concerned.

Sexual disorders

A. SEXUAL DYSFUNCTION

ERECTILE IMPOTENCE

Types
1. *Total*. Neither psychic nor reflexive erections since puberty, or at the most only partial erections have occurred.
2. *Acute onset (primary)*. Erections may have occurred with fantasy or spontaneously but never successful sexual intercourse.
3. *Acute onset (secondary)*. Follows a period of normal potency and often related to traumatic event.
4. *Gradual onset (secondary)*. Following a period of normal potency, there occurs fall off in sexual interest and increasingly frequent erectile failure.

Causes
Type 1 is uncommon, possibly related to constitutional low sex drive. Type 2 and 3 often related to anxiety in sexual situation though may not have neurotic personality. Anxiety causes arousal above optimal for erection to occur when the optimal level is low, or there is negative correlation between arousal and erection. Type 4 has less obvious relation to anxiety which if present may be secondarily related to impotence. Tends to affect older men who have previous history of varying sexual interest. Sexual partner often the prime motivator in seeking treatment.

Psychological factors important in 90%, usually involving anxiety related to perceived threat in the sexual situation (e.g. due to poor sexual education, guilt and fear of discovery, punishment, loss of control, pregnancy). Depressive illness also important. Marked individual variation in cause of impotence related to level of anxiety, type of psychodynamic problem, vulnerability of potency mechanisms.

Secondary relationship difficulties frequently follow and the resulting hostility, estrangement and increased anxiety complicate the problem: attitude of sexual partner then becomes crucial and may be major perpetuating factor.

Organic factors important in 10%. Tend to give picture of persistent, progressive disability in contrast to psychogenic factors which tend to cause more variable disability, often related to specific situations.

Diabetes mellitus a common cause: 30–60% diabetic men have potency disorders. May occur when diabetes out of control; other possible factors include diabetic neuropathy, arteriosclerotic changes in penile vessels, hormonal and biochemical disorder and secondary psychogenesis.

Drugs causing impotence: adrenergic blockers, phenothiazines (especially thioridazine), imipramine (atropine like effects) MAOIs, minor tranquillisers. Alcohol excess a common precipitant.

Chronic debilitating disease, vascular obstruction of lower aorta, prostatectomy (rare and usually there is a preceding history of sexual dysfunction), temporal lobe disorders.

Endocrine disorders: adrenal and thyroid dysfunction.

Male climacteric (low plasma testosterone and high gonadotrophin) a dubious entity. Very uncommon cause of impotence, if at all. Castration, eunuchoidism, Klinefelter's syndrome, infantilism, ingestion of female hormones or antiandrogens. Relation between testosterone and impotence is complex. When impotence due to castration before puberty testosterone causes no improvement. Later onset cases occasionally respond to it but even when blood level of testosterone is initially low there may be little or no improvement.

PREMATURE EJACULATION

Persistent occurrence of ejaculation and orgasm against volition before the male wishes, before or immediately after penetration.

May date from adolescence or may be of later onset.

Sexual drive may be high or low.

May occur independently of erectile impotence or co-exist with it.

DELAYED OR ABSENT EJACULATION

Persistent absence of orgasm and ejaculation during coitus, in spite of normal desire and erection. Occasionally absence of ejaculation only ('dry run' orgasm) which may complicate use of hypotensive and major tranquilliser drugs or prostatectomy.

Delayed orgasm may be related to lack of drive due to sexual deviation or anxiety. May resemble gradual onset impotence with life long sexual hypo-excitability.

VAGINISMUS

Involuntary spasm of circular fibres of levator ani: in severe cases also the adductors of the thigh, erector spinae and glutei when sexual intercourse is attempted by male partner.

Causes. Usually a learnt maladaptive response. Fear of being hurt, possibly related to previous painful experience, long standing fear of intercourse, faulty sex education, sex equated with guilt. Vicious circle of failure, e.g. marital tension, accentuation of any potency problem husband may have.

Assessment. May show acute anxiety on digital vaginal examination.

FRIGIDITY

Impairment of woman's capacity for genital sensory pleasure or for any aspect of the emotional experience coincident with it. May be absence of orgasm, vulval anaesthesia.

Causes. Often but not necessarily reflects wider marital and/or personality problems. May be temporary after childbirth, related to fatigue, physical ill health, anxiety over day to day matters, depression, fear of pregnancy, dislike of contraception, coitus interruptus over prolonged period of time, lack of privacy. Secondary marital tension often perpetuates.

TREATMENT OF SEXUAL DYSFUNCTION

Important to provide adequate treatment for other related disorders.

Drugs
Variable effect of anxiolytics. Androgens of uncertain value in impotence: a small proportion of cases may respond to high dose depot preparation of testosterone e.g. Sustanon 250 mg weekly.

Marital counselling
Use initially when wider conflict in marital relationship is paramount: include non-sexual issues.

Individual psychotherapy
If neurotic personality difficulties severe.

Behaviour therapy
Pioneered by Masters and Johnson who outline the principles of the New Sex Therapy as follows:

Physiological response such as erection, which itself cannot be consciously controlled directly, is not striven for per se: allowed to take care of itself.

Brief highly concentrated behavioural psychotherapy aimed directly at symptoms, e.g. daily sessions for 2 weeks.

The couple seen as a functioning unit through which treatment occurs. Joint responsibility for progress, neither being the primary patient.

Dual-Sex Therapy Team. Important to counter any tendency for one therapist to impose own personal values on the couple: permits fuller understanding of both male and female attitudes: controls any sexual element in transference.

Aim is to give pleasure rather than receive it. Clear goals at all stages.

Sequence in treatment. Basic education (anatomy/physiology) establish good communication, full discussion of sexual feelings, hostilities, resentments.

Sensate focus with ban on intercourse or genital contact. Mutual exploration to establish areas of pleasurable tactile stimulation. Primary aim is not own sexual gratification, couple freed from demands of responding sexually, and so 'performance fears' reduced. These lead to loss of spontaneity, a tendency to watch own performance (spectator role) and to self-validating fears when partner is seen to become less spontaneous.

Specific dysfunction dealt with after sensate focus established. In impotence allow female to play dominant role, avoid sudden switch from foreplay to intercourse. In premature ejaculation female masturbates partner to point just short of ejaculation, then squeezes glans between thumb and first two fingers (Seman's technique). Gradual assumption of sexual intercourse. Vaginismus may require initial relaxation and individual psychotherapy (may include use of dilators) before couple therapy can proceed.

PROGNOSIS IN SEXUAL DYSFUNCTION

Good outcome associated with previous adequate sexual function, acute onset impotence, short duration of disability, adequate heterosexual desire, free from other psychological problems, and absence of secondary estrangement.

B. SEXUAL DEVIATION

DEFINITIONS

Anomaly of sexual inclination and behaviour which is not part of a psychosis or other illness.

Homosexuality. Sexual attraction with or without physical relationship between members of the same sex.

Fetishism. Sexual excitation and gratification arises mainly or exclusively from inanimate articles somehow related to the human body usually of the opposite sex, often articles of clothing.

Paedophilia. Desire of adult to engage in sexual activity with children of either sex.

Transvestism. Sexual pleasure derived from dressing and sometimes masquerading in clothing of opposite sex.

Exhibitionism. Sexual gratification from exposure of the male genitals to females.

HOMOSEXUALITY IN THE MALE

37% males experience orgasm during homosexual behaviour at some time. (Kinsey U.S.A. 1948.)

Common, even regarded as normal in societies which do not prohibit it.

May be transient phase in adolescence.

Causes

Those that push individual away from heterosexuality.
Learnt inhibition (family attitudes, ignorance, fear of disease).
Incestuous feelings about mother or sisters.
Lack of confidence in own sexual potency, sexual identity.

Those that pull towards homosexuality
Need for security may dominate any sensual aspect of relationship especially when older male chosen.
Self esteem when not available through other relationship.
Fear of males causes erotic passive response (ethological parallels).
Material gain.

Congenital and prenatal
Increased concordance rates in twins (same incidence in MZ and DZ pairs).
Presence of androgen at critical pre and neonatal periods determine later masculine type of behaviour.

Environmental factors
Probably predominate in choice of gender identity. Abnormal relationship with parents: unsatisfactory or absent relationship with father. Close binding intimate relationship with mother who may behave erotically towards son, prefer him to husband, overprotect and discourage his normal heterosexual development.

Choice of regular homosexual identity may be related to secondary perpetuating factors which depend on how rewarding it continues to be. May retain both heterosexual and homosexual orientation. Latter may then be source of marked anxiety. Others completely identify with homosexual identity and adopt mannerisms and life style accordingly, ensuring its perpetuation.

Management
Establish clear aims and reasons for referral. Coercion not justified.
   Treat concomitant problems (mood disorders, neurotic illness,
social support). May prefer to continue with homosexual
orientation: support accordingly.
   Those who wish to become heterosexual; true motivation for
change crucial and the amount of coercion from other must be
evaluated.
   Treatment focussed on four main areas: reduction of
heterosexual anxiety, increase in heterosexual responsiveness,
development of satisfactory heterosexual behaviour, reduction of
deviant sexual interest.
   40% show benefit from treatment.

Specialised techniques
Indication of good response include age less than 35 years, and the
presence of some heterosexual interest at some stage in the past,
absence of widespread personality difficulties and perpetuating
attitudes. Treatment must be combined with regular review
discussions.
   Systematic desensitisation more effective than aversion in those
who have obvious heterosexual anxiety. Aversion more effective
when less general anxiety but some anxiety about homosexuality.
   Encourage adoption of heterosexual social interaction and
behaviour, in paralled with specific behaviour therapy. Other
psychological difficulties may appear during treatment e.g.
depression, difficulty in relinquishing life style, realisation that
sexual deviance has led to secondary gain (e.g. avoidance of social
situation in social phobia).
   Techniques of modification: aversion therapy involves
association of noxious stimulus (emetics to produce nausea,
electrical stimuli), with deviant stimuli or responses either mental
or physiological (e.g. penile erection).
   Modification of sexual fantasies by pairing them with imagined
unpleasant mental images and by encouraging heterosexual
masturbatory images.
   Systematic desensitisation used when marked anxiety towards
heterosexual situation present. Progression through hierarchy with
relaxation. May involve Masters and Johnson principles.
   Positive conditioning of sexual reponse using pleasant reward.

HOMOSEXUALITY IN THE FEMALE

2.2% of adult female population (England and Wales). Kinsey found
4% single women remained exclusively lesbian from 20–35 years
of age. More often related to companionship than sexual
gratification. Lesbian relationships tend to be more stable than

those between homosexual males. Increased vulnerability to episodes of depression, anxiety.

EXHIBITIONISM

Accounts for one third of all recidivist sexual offenders. Rarely associated with indecent assault or sexual violence. May signify increased risk of paedophilia or hebephilic tendencies, homosexual contact and voyeurism.

Not a clear cut syndrome: part of behaviour dominated by immature goals of genital display, inspection and manipulation. Tend to be timid and unassertive socially, though aggressive in own family. Suggest disorder in ability to handle and express aggressive impulses. Often complain of impotence, premature ejaculation.

TRANS SEXUALISM

The wish to change sex, often with deep conviction that assignment to wrong sex has occurred.

Sustained feminine gender identification and wish to alter bodily appearance towards opposite sex.

Some heterosexual drive likely to be present if there has been a history of fetishistic arousal.

More common in men than in women. Passive homosexual male may seek sex reassignment to rationalise a relationship. 47XYY genotype may predispose to trans sexualism.

TRANSVESTISM

The wish to wear clothing appropriate to the opposite sex, often associated with sexual gratification. Some resemblance to fetishism. Heterosexual drive predominates in 67%; homosexual in 33%.

Psychotherapy useful in supportive form but relatively ineffective in achieving radical change in sex orientation. Hormone therapy (oestrogens, antiandrogens in male). Aversion therapy possibly more effective in transvestism than in trans sexualism.

Sex reassignment surgery. Used in a small minority of trans sexualism (single, absence of antisocial behaviour, intelligent enough to adapt to change, over 21, must have irrevocable pattern of cross-sex behaviour).

INTERSEXUALITY

A state between normal male and normal female.

Causes
Chromosomal. (Turner's syndrome, triple X female, chromatin
positive Klinefelter's syndrome 47XXY, double Y male 47XYY.
   Gonadal. (True hermaphroditism with both ovaries and testes,
simple gonadal dysgenesis.)
   Mullerian. (Disordered embryogenesis.)
   Hormonal. (Adrenal hyperplasia at birth or later causing
virilisation in female; early failure of foetal testes or failed response
of target organ to androgens may cause feminisation in male. May
also be due to tumours of testes, adrenal or pituitary glands, liver
disease, administration of oestrogen.)
   Diagnosis of sex at birth: apparent sex judged by genitalia (may
be deceptive), nuclear sex (females have chromocentric or Barr body
indicating 2 X chromosomes in buccal smear) chromosome
analysis, urinary 17 ketosteroids.

SEXUAL OFFENDERS

Tend to be older than other offenders and to be of slightly lower
intelligence. Recent increase in number of adolescent indecent
exposers. Victim may play part in initiating episode and dictate its
precise form by her subsequent reaction.

Exhibitionism
3000 convictions in England and Wales per annum. Rate doubled
since World War 2 though that for adult men constant. Group
therapy may help shy passive individuals. Systematic
desensitisation of heterosexual anxiety also useful.

Rape
Sexual intercourse with a woman against her will whether by force,
fraud or intimidation. More than one third occur between
acquaintances. Motives may range from misunderstanding in
sexual situation to deeper hostility towards females.
   May require prolonged psychotherapy: group setting may be
helpful. Hormone therapy when sex drive extreme.

Paedophilia
Children under 16 years not legally capable of giving sexual
consent. (A man cannot give consent to homosexual act if under 21
years). Psychotherapy, especially group, behaviour therapy. In
extreme cases hormone therapy.

Incest
Prior to 1908 this was not a criminal offence. Incestuous father may
merely disregard normal sexual taboos, may be paedophiliac or
may have other sexual psychopathology. Whole family may need
to be treated.

Sexual violence
A proportion (22%) of long term prisoners have committed offence involving some kind of overt sexual activity. Tend to be more violent than remainder, though less recidivist.

Treatment of sexual offenders
Hormone therapy. Patient must be fully informed of risks and given signed consent. Needs to be well motivated, and only justified in disorders liable to cause serious social complications. Oestrogens may cause breast hypertrophy, testicular atrophy, osteoporosis (oral ethinyl oestradiol 0.01 – 0.05 mg/day causes least nausea). Depot preparation: oestradiol undecylenate 50 – 100mg once every 3 – 4 weeks. Benperidol or butyrophenone and the antiandrogen cyproterone acetate also used.

Where possible treatment should be as a condition of probation. Criminal Justice Act 1972 allows this kind of treatment for up to 3 years, the patient remaining in the community.

FURTHER READING

SEXUAL DEVIATION

Armstrong, C. N. (1968) Intersexuality. *Brit. J. Hosp. Med.* March 667 – 673.
Bancroft, J. H. J. (1974) *Deviant Sexual Behaviour.* Oxford: Clarendon Press.
Gunn, J. (1976) Sexual offenders. *Brit. J. Hosp. Med.* Jan., 57 – 65.
Randell, J. (1970) Transvestism and trans sexualism. *Brit. J. Hosp. Med.* Feb., 211 – 213.
Rooth, G. (1973) Exhibitionism, sexual violence and paedophilia. *Brit. J. Psychiat.*, **122**, 705 – 710.

SEXUAL DYSFUNCTION

Bancroft, J. H. J. (1970) Disorders of sexual potency. In *Modern Trends in Psychosomatic Medicine 2*, ed. O. W. Hill. London: Butterworths.
Bancroft, J. H. J. Sexual dysfunction in men. *Medicine*, **30**, 1790 – 1792.
Cooper, A. J. (1970) Male sex dysfunction. *Brit. Med. J.*, **1**, 157 – 159.
Cooper, A. J. (1972) Endocrine impotence. *Brit. Med. J.*, **2**, 34 – 36.
Masters, W. H. & Johnson, V. E. (1970) *Human Sexual Inadequacy.* Boston: Little, Brown.
Masters, W. H. & Johnson, V. E. (1976) Principles of the new sex therapy. *Am. J. Psychiat.*, **133**, 548 – 554.
Spencer, E. Psychosexual problems in women. *Medicine*, **30**, 1793 – 1796.

Alcoholism

DEFINITIONS

Abnormal dependence a central concept. Initially this may be entirely psychological but it later progresses to physical dependence (i.e. true addiction) with biochemical changes at cellular level leading to withdrawal symptoms when alcohol intake reduced.

WHO (1952)
Alcoholics are those excessive drinkers whose dependence on alcohol has attained such a degree that it shows noticeable disturbance or an interference with their bodily and mental health, their personal relationships, and smooth economic functioning, or who show prodomal signs of such a development. They therefore need treatment.

Jellinek (1960)
. . . 'any use of alcoholic beverages that cause any damage to the individual or society or both'.

Chafetz (1974)
. . . 'any drinking behaviour that is associated with dysfunction in a person's life'.
   Such definitions can be difficult to apply because the concept of disease entity is ill-defined, and they do not clearly delineate social from morbid use of alcohol. Addiction and harm are not synonymous: harm may occur without addiction, and true addiction may exist without obvious harm for long periods. Davies (1971) suggests definition of alcoholism as 'the intermittent or continual ingestion of alcohol leading to dependency (addiction) or harm.'

EPIDEMIOLOGY

Prevalence
Early case detection difficult (failure of others to recognise, patient denial). About 400 000–700 000 alcoholics in U.K. (15–20 per G.P.)

If include relatives, 1 in 25 closely affected by this illness (1 in 10 in Scotland and Northern Ireland).

Hospital admission statistics (England and Wales)
First admission: primary diagnosis alcoholism or alcoholic psychosis

1949	*1952*	*1972*
434	2000	10 167

Partly related to increased services, though consistent with rise according to other indices such as the national drink bill, number of drunkenness convictions. Prevalence of alcohol cirrhosis increased by 163% since 1963. During the 1970s, deaths from cirrhosis and alcoholism both increased by 30%, and driving offences related to alcohol more than doubled. 1 in 3 drivers killed had excess blood alcohol.

Jellinek Formula $A = R(PD/K)$ where D = no. of deaths from cirrhosis, A = prevalence of severe alcoholism, P = proportion of cirrhotic deaths due to alcoholism, K = constant (0.695) derived from $C_1C_2/100(C_1$ being % of alcoholics with cirrhosis, C_2 being % mortality among alcoholics with cirrhosis).

The formula estimates prevalence in England + Wales of 11/1000 general population though it has been criticised because K changes with time and varies from one community to another.

Prevalence surveys

	per 1000 gen. popn.			
	Male	*Female*	*Total*	
Medical & community agencies	6.2	1.4		Moss, Beresford, Davies
General practitioners			1.1	Parr
			2.0	Shepherd
			10.2	Wilkins

The more recent Wilkins survey included problem drinkers plus addicts, in central Manchester (high density population) and involved direct interviews with persons possessing 'at risk' characteristics who attended G.P.s.

Cohort studies	*Life expectancy of alcoholism*
Iceland (Helgason)	6–10% male; 0.4% female
Bornholm (Fremming)	3.4% male; 0.1% female

Interviews with representative sample of population (Manhatten U.S.A.) Prevalence 19/1000.

Of medical admissions to hospitals in U.K.: 18% (Moody 1976). in U.S.A.: 21–41% (Tamayo and Feldman 1978).

Sex
Male/Female ratio 4.3:1 (females may be detected less easily, and probably increasing incidence).

Age
Recent marked increase in young adults in Scotland.

Social class
In U.K. high in Class 1 in which cirrhosis also most common. In Italy, Sweden, some parts U.S.A., most common in lower social classes. Lowest prevalence normally in middle class.

Occupation
High morbidity when there is ease of access to alcohol and its use is condoned. Morbidity increased X 9 in trade representatives of alcohol manufacturers and distributors. Special hazard in armed forces.

Ethnic group
High in Irish and North American Negro. Low in Jews.

Marital status
High in divorced, separated, widowers.

National alcohol intake
Correlates with higher prevalence in France than in Italy.

Living conditions
Higher prevalence in urban than rural especially high living density.

CLINICAL FEATURES

Problem drinking
Arises out of social drinking. Great variation. Before onset of physical dependence. Usually presents with social, interpersonal, work, economic difficulties. Existence becomes increasingly centred around alcohol, ensuring its availability. Increased alcohol intake, especially symptomatic drinking at times of stress, and surreptitious intake. May be episodes of acute drunkenness. Physical symptoms: anorexia, nausea, diarrhoea, retching, especially in mornings. Psychological symptoms: anxiety, depression, transient reversible memory lapses for recent events (palimpsests), denial, rationalisation, projection, regarding alcohol use. Resent discussing it.

Addictive drinking
Jellinek distinguished 5 patterns of pathological drinking:
α purely psychological dependence to relieve bodily or emotional

pain. No loss of control (i.e. able to curtail amount taken).
β physiological complications e.g. cirrhosis but no dependence.
γ loss of control, common in spirit drinkers. Can abstain.
θ High tissue tolerance and withdrawal symptoms when attempt to abstain. Otherwise may show no social disruption from drinking.
ε spree drinking.

Jellinek saw addiction as loss of control and/or inability to abstain.

This classification criticised: deterioration through these categories not inevitable. Loss of control a variable phenomenon and may depend on availability of alcohol. It is not inevitable each time alcohol is taken, and it is difficult to predict which drinking episode will precipitate it.

NATURAL HISTORY OF ADDICTION (untreated)

(Lemere quoted by Edwards 1967)
28% drink themselves to death.
10% regain some control.
29% continue to have life long problem.
22% stop in a terminal illness.
11% stop spontaneously.

COMPLICATIONS OF ADDICTION

Acute drunkenness
Highly likely when blood alcohol level more than 100 mg %. Some variation with level of tissue tolerance and rate of gut absorption depending on other stomach contents. More likely when some degree of brain damage present. Potentiated by other drugs such as barbiturates. If comatose, remember that this may be due to some other cause even though patient may smell of alcohol, and may be due to alcohol even when there is no smell of it.

Withdrawal symptoms
Onset 0–8 hours. Tremor, nausea, retching, sweating, vivid anxiety-provoking dreams. May proceed to delirium tremens (see below).

Alcohol tolerance
Initially increased, later impaired.

Psychological
Angry outbursts, disinhibited behaviour. Defence mechanisms. Anxiety, depression.

Deliberate self harm, either non fatal or suicide. The latter increased × 80 in male alcoholics (Kessel & Grossman). 16% life expectancy of suicide (Helgason).

Cerebral atrophy: 70% may have radiological evidence especially frontal and parietal lobes. Detectable by psychometric tests in 58%.

Delirium tremens. 48–72 hours after alcohol withdrawal, confusion, disorientation, gross ataxia, agitation, intense fear, visual/tactile hallucinations, paranoid ideation. Usually precipitated by relative or absolute alcohol withdrawal: concurrent infection common. Minor hallucinatory symptoms complicate withdrawal in 50% alcohol addicts, full blown DTs in 5%. Mortality from this 15% (infection, dehydration, injury, hyperthermia, circulatory collapse, status epilepticus).

Alcoholic auditory hallucinosis: may be part of withdrawal syndrome, but may be independent of this, in setting of clear consciousness. Most last few days, a few become chronic. Uncertain relationship to incipient schizophrenia or dementia.

Wernicke's encephalopathy: confusion, ataxia, nystagmus, internuclear ophthalmoplegia, disorder of conjugate gaze. Probably due to thiamine deficiency, acute degenerative changes in mammillary bodies, mid brain, brain stem. May lead to Korsakoff's psychosis with gross impairment of new learning and retention of very recent memory, occasionally complicated by confabulation.

Morbid jealousy. May be related to impotence, rejection by partner.

Physical
Mortality 113% greater than expected. Increased incidence of respiratory disease, gastritis, peptic ulcer, pancreatitis, accidents, vascular disease (? related to hypertriglyceridaemia) neoplasms of larynx and upper digestive tracts, cardiomyopathy and heart failure. Nutritional deficiency, especially Vitamin B1. Early obesity, later weight loss.

Liver metabolism. Coenzyme NAD becomes reduced by alcohol dehydrogenase leading to rise in lactic and ketoacids. Acetaldehyde may be the cause of mitochondrial swelling after acute alcohol ingestion. Increased microsomal enzyme activity. Impaired gluconeogenesis (may cause hypoglycaemia after alcohol intake, usually when glycogen depleted). Reduced albumin and transferrin synthesis, increased lipoprotein synthesis, decreased fatty acid oxidation (fatty infiltration).

Alcoholic hepatitis. Usually after long history (10 years) alcohol abuse, precipitated by acute intoxication. Acute illness resembling viral hepatitis (pain, fever, jaundice), 10–30% die in hepatic failure, others may develop cirrhosis.

Cirrhosis. Hepatic fibrosis at early stage leading to portal hypertension. Occurs in 5–10% chronic alcoholics. 65% of all cases of cirrhosis are related to alcohol abuse. May develop encephalopathy (precipitated by haemorrhage, infection, sedatives, surgical procedures, protein intake). Oesophageal varices may be a major problem.

Neurological. Head injury, epilepsy, poly neuropathy, (tender calves, impaired tendon reflexes, muscle wasting, sensory loss, unpleasant dysaesthesiae: probably caused by combined toxic effect of alcohol and nutritional deficiency), acute cerebellar degeneration, central pontine myelinoclisis (bulbar palsy, spastic quadriparesis, usually rapidly fatal). Marchiafava Bignamy disease (intellectual impairment, fits, pyramidal signs, degeneration of corpus callosum) myopathy (acute or subacute with proximal muscle weakness), optic atrophy (methyl alcohol intake).

Foetal alcohol syndrome. Prenatal damage related to heavy alcohol intake by mother during pregnancy. Poor growth (67%), impaired intellectual development, facial changes, congenital defects 30–40%, neonatal mortality 17% (Hanson).

Family
Marital discord and failure. Children of alcoholic parents: increased risk of becoming alcoholic themselves later, marrying an alcoholic, developing other psychiatric problems. Alcoholics' wives: described as dominant, aggressive, masochistic, but no adequate control studies on this. Difficult to distinguish behaviour secondary to alcoholism in spouse from that which antedates it. Wives have increased incidence of alcoholism in own parents, and may have married an alcoholic previously (? selective mating in some marriages). Occasionally connive with husband's drinking and in denying it. She may develop problems when husband becomes sober.

CAUSES

Social
Ethnic variation related to group attitudes as well as individual characteristics. Protection by identification of alcohol with religious ritual (Jews). Relevant factors: degree of group anxiety and acculturation, lack of social hierarchy or of alternative means of satisfaction.

Predisposing attitudes: alcohol use equated with masculinity, group solidarity and relaxation (as opposed to use with meals), symptomatic problem-solving use, ambivalent community attitude to alcohol.

National economic pressure: in France where many involved in alcohol trade the level of acceptable alcohol consumption high.

Personal
Genetic. High concordance in MZ twins (54.2% compared with 31% DZ), may be related to personality traits rather than specific genetic

factors. No demonstrable antecedent metabolic defect
demonstrated.

Psychological. Learnt habit: imitation, operant learning (social
reward of anxiety reduction or prevention), classical conditioning
(Orford 1971). Imitation, identification may be relevant to increased
vulnerability in children of alcoholic parents.

Personality: no single type. Often dependent, passive or anxiety
prone.

TREATMENT

Early recognition: avoid stereotype of deterioration as synonymous
with alcoholism.

'At risk' factors in patients attending G.P.s and probability of
being alcoholic (Wilkins): 100% if previous drunkenness offence or
ask for help with alcohol problem, 75% if smell of drink at
consultation, 50% if peptic ulcer, gastritis, request sick note for
symptoms which do not suggest physical illness, accident at home,
live in hostel for homeless, 25% if work in catering or brewery
trade, divorced or separated, single male over 40 years, history of
marital dysharmony (Central Manchester).

Motivation: facilitate by education on effects of alcohol,
confrontation, (e.g. ability to abstain), support, reassure and convey
conviction that recovery possible, set realistic goals. Ultimate
strategy may require removal of support which perpetuates
pathological drinking.

The setting: out-patient management may be sufficient in two
thirds of cases. In-patient treatment may be needed when
withdrawal symptoms severe. Short stay (3 weeks) may be as
effective as longer stay.

Detoxification centres in experimental stage in U.K. attempt to
provide alternative to ineffective convictions for drunkenness.
Referrals by police of persons drunk in public places.

Withdrawal symptoms: may need sedatives (chlordiazepoxide,
chlormethiazole). Important to treat fluid, electrolyte and nutritional
deficiencies. May need infusion of glucose and Vit. B. Watch for
infection, prevent injury. Use anticonvulsants if fits occur, or
previous history of these. Magnesium used by some centres to
reduce CNS excitability.

The addiction: individual, group, conjoint, family therapy.
Commitment of therapist crucial. Previous claims of aversion
therapy (apormorphine, emetine difficult to evaluate (patient
selection, high cost treatment). Antabuse useful in preventing
impending relapse: reactions can be dangerous. Best to aim at total
abstinence. Brief counselling may be as effective as prolonged
therapy (Orford & Edwards).

Return to controlled social drinking: unlikely to succeed if
physical addiction has been present.

Community services crucial: information centres and Councils on Alcoholism, hostels, social services, alcohol programmes in industry. Alcoholics Anonymous: mutual group supportive help emphasises cohesiveness, helping others, sharing of information and hope.

Prevention: Education on responsible use of alcohol, cost control of alcoholic drinks, responsible advertising, judicious use of restricted availability.

GOOD PROGNOSTIC FACTORS

Social stability, older, male, absence of psychopathic traits, cooperative attitude, amenable to change, first treatment, adequate intelligence.

FURTHER READING

Davies, D. L. (1971) Alcoholism. *Update*, July, 885–888.
Edwards, G. (1967) The meaning and treatment of alcohol dependence. *Brit. J. Hosp. Med.*, Dec., 272–281.
Glatt, M. M. (1974) Alcoholism. Brit. J. Hosp. Med., Jan. 111–120.
Hore, B. D. (1976) *Alcohol Dependence*. London: Butterworths.
Moody, P. M. (1976) Drinking and smoking behaviour of hospitalised medical patients. *J. Stud. Alc.*, **37**, 1317–1319.
Orford, J. (1971) Psychological approaches to alcoholism. *Update*, Aug., p. 1005.
Orford, J. (1974) Alcoholism and marriage: the argument against specialism. *J. Stud. Alc.*, **36**, 1537.
Orford, 1. & Edwards, G. (1977) *Alcoholism*. Maudsley Monograph No. 26. London: Oxford University Press.
Royal College of Psychiatrists (1979) *Alcohol and alcoholism. The report of a special committee.* London: Tavistock
Tamayo, M. B. & Feldman, D. J. (1975) Incidence of alcoholism in hospital patients. *Social Wk. N.Y.*, **20**, 89–91.
See *Brit. J. Hosp. Med.*, Aug. 1977 for articles on clinical features, liver, neurological, cardiac and foetal complications.

Drug addiction

DEFINITION

WHO (1969): a state, psychic and sometimes also physical, resulting from the interaction between a living organism and a drug, characterised by behavioural and other responses that always include a compulsion to take the drug on a continuous or periodic basis in order to experience its psychic effects and sometimes to avoid the discomfort of its absence. Tolerance may or may not be present. A person may be dependent on more than one drug.

LEGISLATION

Misuse of Drugs Act 1971
Controls the import, export, supply, production and possession of certain drugs. Its Advisory Council monitors the national situation and can advise change in categorisation of any drug.

Distinguishes 3 classes of controlled drugs:
a. Includes opium, heroin, morphine, most opiates, pethidine, LSD, mescaline, other hallucinogens, methadone, cocaine, cannabinol, except cannabis resin or cannabis.
b. Includes cannabis and its resin, amphetamine, d. amphetamine.
c. Methaqualone, benzphetamine.

Penalties for abuse
In Magistrates Court:
    Class (a) up to one year imprisonment or £400 fine or both.
    Class (b) six months imprisonment or £400 fine or both.
    Class (c) six months imprisonment or £200 fine or both.
In Crown Court:
    Class (a) up to seven years imprisonment.
    Class (b) up to five years.
    Class (c) up to two years.

Penalty for intent to supply or produce Class (a) or (b) up to 14 years imprisonment.

Misuse of Drugs Regulations 1973
Notification of and Supply to Addicts
Drugs are dealt with in the four schedules. The regulations specify controls in the way more than 100 drugs in schedules two and three may be supplied to addicts. They require that the total quantity, or the number of dosage units should be specified both in words and figures. N.B. Drugs such as amphetamines and methaqualone, methyphenidate, phenmetrazine are subject to the same controls as opiates.

Require notification within 7 days by a doctor to the Chief Medical Officer, Home Office, of any person he has attended who is addicted to dextromoramide, diamorphine, dipipanone, hydrocodone, hydromorphone, levorphanol, methadone, morphine, opium, oxycodone, pethidine, phenazocine, piritramide.

Special licence required before a doctor can prescribe heroin, morphine, cocaine or any of their salts for treatment of addiction.

EPIDEMIOLOGY

Prior to the 1960s opiate dependence in the U.K. limited to relatively few who had been initiated through therapeutic contact with drug.

In 1960s explosive increase occurred in numbers who were addicted to heroin and cocaine, particularly in Metropolitan London. 500% increase by 1965. Younger persons, not initiated through therapeutic exposure. Social infection. Since then the total problem has continued to increase in size mainly as methadone misuse. Reduction in numbers using heroin, cocaine and other opiates.

Number of addicts known to Home Office

	1970	1975
TOTAL	1426	1954
Heroin	991	316
Cocaine	57	23
Methadone	991	1543

In 1976 a fall in total occurred (1881) but the number of new notifications 7% higher than in 1975.

Reliability of statistics appears poor because of failure to notify (up to 64% of cases). Inadequate clinical assessment and reluctance to diagnose addiction common.

Most cases of opiate misuse aged 20–30 years, in which group the steepest increase in incidence has occurred. Male/female ratio 3 : 1. Trend towards increasing age of addicts in recent years.

Stereotype of the 'junkie' opiate dependent: social drop out, unemployed, preceding severe personality difficulties. Important to remember that this is the hard core of the problem: many probably use opiates only occasionally without social deterioration (chippers). Up to one third may eventually spontaneously stop drug misuse (Stimson)

Trend towards multiple drug misuse, for example a combination of barbiturates with opiates.

Use of cannabis widespread by young, middle class, above average educational attainment, perhaps leading normal lives without social misfit or psychological instability. Very different from the 'junkie' stereotype and without obvious immediate adverse effects (Plant).

Attenders at drug treatment centres often use opiates from illegal sources as well as from prescription. Thefts from retail chemists have become a major problem. Dipipanone (Diconal) abuse has increased progressively in recent years: proportion of addicts receiving it on prescription 2% in 1974, 6% in 1975 and 8% in 1976.

Increased mortality in young adults ($\times$ 28 expected) mainly related to intravenous misuse, usually involving opiates and barbiturates: may be due to drug overdose (accidental and related to loss of tissue tolerance, or deliberate and suicidal). Other indirect causes not involving lethal overdose also important (traffic or other accident, inhalation of vomit, burns, or in 5% septicaemia).

OPIATES (MORPHINE TYPE)

Now most commonly involves methadone, less often heroin. Cocaine may be used at the same time as a CNS stimulant though it does not produce tolerance effects. Intravenous administration of opiates common leading to marked physical dependence and tolerance and high dosage e.g. 300 mg of heroin per day.

In assessment important to search for injection marks and to carry out full physical examination. Frequently omitted.

Complications
Withdrawal symptoms. Craving, rhinorrhoea, agitation, perspiration, tremor, diarrhoea, tachycardia.

Acute overdosage perhaps leading to coma, (accidental or suicidal).

Infection. Phlebitis, septicaemia, acute bacterial endocarditis (beware recent onset cardiac murmurs), homologous serum jaundice.

Cocaine abuse may cause paranoid state with hallucinations, visual or auditory, intense itching, tactile hallucinations of insects crawling on skin (formication).

Causes
Under-privileged background common with history of marked under-achievement. Resolution of frustration by developing group solidarity with others who are similar (Plant).

Management

Overdose. As for any coma. Nalorphine may precipitate severe withdrawal symptoms. Beware of ventricular fibrillation if cocaine is involved.

Withdrawal symptoms. May be controlled by oral methadone (as linctus) 10 mg initially, repeat 20 mg 1 hour later if no improvement. Maximum 50 mg in 12 hours. Beware of withdrawal fits when barbiturates abused also.

Treatment of the addiction
In the U.K. maintenance therapy permitted. Contrast U.S.A. where opiate addiction is regarded as criminal. Oral methadone preferable. Regular urine drug assay crucial. Current approach increasingly conservative and opiates used in treatment only as last resort for specific period of time. Need to monitor whether this approach will lead to increase in illicit misuse of drugs. Intensive support over long periods essential in rehabilitation.

BARBITURATES

Increasing incidence, often involving intravenous route. Can cause necrotic skin ulcers. May be part of multiple drug abuse. Overdose leads to ataxia, dysarthria and dangerous coma. Withdrawal symptoms similar to alcohol when physical dependence is present: tremor, hallucinatory confusional state, akin to delirium tremens, fits. Drug withdrawal best carried out gradually in physically dependent individuals.

AMPHETAMINES

Cause stimulation, increased energy, euphoria, aggressive behaviour. Prolonged heavy abuse (more than 50 mg per day) may lead to paranoid hallucinatory schizophrenic-like psychosis: usually resolved when drug stopped, but occasionally becomes chronic. Withdrawal may be complicated by severe depression and suicidal risk. Methyl amphetamine often abused intravenously: vivid visual hallucinations common.

LSD

Not accompanied by dependence. Adverse effects include paranoid hallucinatory psychosis, acute anxiety, confusion, impaired judgement, disorientation. Recurrence may occur some weeks after intake stopped. Uncertain whether it can cause chronic psychosis. Chlorpromazine useful in severe reactions.

MARIHUANA (CANNABIS)

Widespread casual recreational use. No physical dependence. Causes euphoria, relaxation and sedation. Effects may occasionally be adverse, including depression, panic, distorted time perception, hallucinations, increased auditory acuity. These probably more common in vulnerable personalities but they are unpredictable. May lead to errors of judgement, for example in driving. Users of marijuana are in general hostile to opiate abuse.

NICOTINE

Psychological and physiological dependence.

Types
Psychosocial (little nicotine intake and intermittent).
Indulgent (pleasurable oral reward).
Tranquillisation (usage often varies with emotional state).
Stimulation (to allay fatigue and maintain performance).
Addictive (to avoid withdrawal symptoms and maintain high levels of nicotine in the blood).

MISCELLANEOUS

Wide variety of drugs may become the subject of addictive misuse and constant surveillance required. Glue sniffing a recent example: may be complicated by liver damage.

FURTHER READING

Bewley, T. H. (1970) An introduction to drug dependence. *Brit. J. Hosp. Med.* August, 150–161.
Cahal, D. A. (1974) Misuse of Drugs Act. *Brit. Med. J.*, **1**, 70–72, 73–75.
DHSS (1977) *Advisory Council on the Misuse of Drugs: First Interim Report.*
Granville-Grossman, K. (1971) Drug dependence. In *Recent Advances in Clinical Psychiatry–1*. Edinburgh: Churchill Livingstone.
Plant, M. A. (1974) What is the drug problem? *Social Work Today*, **5**, 277–279.
Russell, M. A. H. (1971) Cigarette dependence. *Brit. Med J.*, **2**., 330–331.
Stevens, B. C. (1978) Deaths of drug addicts in London, 1970–1974. *Med. Sci. Law*, **18**, 128–137.

Mental subnormality (mental handicap)

DEFINITIONS

A condition of arrested mental development, to be distinguished from dementia in which deterioration from a previously higher level of intellectual function has occurred.

Subnormality
A state of arrested or incomplete development of mind, which includes subnormality of intelligence and is of a nature or degree which requires or is susceptible to medical treatment or other special care or training.

Severe subnormality
Renders the person incapable of living an independent life or of guarding himself against serious exploitation, or will be so incapable when of an age to do so.
   These definitions emphasise general personality and social functioning rather than I.Q. though subnormality tends to correspond to an I.Q. range of 50–75 and severe subnormality an I.Q. below 50.
   Mental subnormality is relevant to the Mental Health Act 1983 only if it leads to mental impairment (see p. 93).

PREVALENCE

Severe subnormality
Prevalence 3.6/1000 general population. Usually declared at early age, unable to acquire reading or writing.

Subnormality
Prevalence more difficult to determine: criteria such as employability unreliable (dependent on local economic conditions). 2–3% of population have I.Q. less than 70.

CAUSES

Severe subnormality
Usually secondary to gross organic defects in central nervous system due to following causes:

Genetic
   Autosomal dominant gene (e.g. tuberose sclerosis). 50% of subsequent children are likely to stand at risk of inheriting the gene and therefore being affected unless the gene has arisen *de novo* as a new mutation. This is the case in 80–90% of patients with tuberose sclerosis. When this occurs, subsequent children born to parents do not stand at increased risk.

   Autosomal recessive gene. Each parent is a clinically normal carrier. Theoretical chance that 25% of children will be affected (homozygous): 50% will be normal carriers (heterozygous): 25% will be normal and completely free from the gene. Consanguineous mating important predisposing factor.

   Sex-linked recessive gene. Males usually affected. Females normal carriers. If mother is a carrier then approximately 50% of her progeny are likely to inherit the gene: of these males will be affected; the females carriers.

   Chromosomal. Trisomy 21 mongolism, XXY Klinefelter.

Intrauterine
Infective (rubella, syphilis, toxoplasmosis), metabolic (cretinism, kernicterus due to Rhesus incompatibility), anoxic (ante partum haemorrhage).

At birth, infancy, childhood
Traumatic (brain injury including nonaccidental type), infective (meningitis, encephalitis), anoxic, severe prematurity.

Idiopathic
Probably the largest group. May be associated with gross anatomical CNS defects such as hydrocephalus, microcephaly.

Subnormality
Not so commonly associated with organic CNS defects.
   In less severe forms it is a variation of the normal distribution of mental ability.
   All causes of severe subnormality relevant.
   Social conditions causing lack of educational stimulus, may lead to apparent mild subnormality which is susceptible to improvement.

Subnormality not associated with brain damage is far more common in lower social classes: this has been termed the subcultural type or educationally subnormal, probably directly due to social factors, and preventable.

CLINICAL FEATURES

The severely subnormal child does not acquire reading or writing. May need hospitalisation to ensure adequate level of care and prevent self injury.
Ability to survive in community related to general personality development, especially affective warmth, as well as intellectual level.
Mild subnormality may cause little functional impairment.
Secondary disability as reaction to handicap (e.g. emotional upset, aggressive behaviour) may be precipitated by educational misplacement.
Family may also show emotional upset caused by management difficulties.
Complications: failure in self care, antisocial behaviour (lack of moral sense, aggressive outbursts, especially when over-stressed or frustrated) exploitation by others, prostitution.

INVESTIGATIONS

In infancy. Recognition and vigorous treatment of rhesus incompatibility and infections. Metabolic screening. Clinical assessment permits early recognition of mongolism.
    School children. Regular assessment of intellectual capacity.
    Differentiate from: childhood autism and psychosis, deafness, visual impairment and developmental aphasia.
    The heterozygotes for some autosomal recessive conditions (e.g. phenylketonuria) in most cases can be detected by biochemical and specific enzyme assay techniques. This may involve assay of fetal cells obtained by amniocentesis. Parents who have already had a child with such a disorder should be alerted to the availability of prenatal diagnosis in subsequent pregnancies. Similar considerations apply to sex-linked recessive conditions such as Lesch-Nyhan and Hunter's syndromes in which heterozygotes (female carriers) can be identified by specific enzyme assay of cells. The sex of the fetus can be determined by chromosome investigation: termination of pregnancy may be offered when an affected male fetus is identified.

MANAGEMENT

Prevention
Genetic counselling, good obstetric and child care.
Early detection of parents liable to cause non-accidental injury.

Treatment
Should emphasise individual care and interpersonal contact.
Adequate opportunity and stimulus.
Small family-type units as opposed to custodial regimes.
Care in community preferable to institutional.
Day centre and training scheme integrated with local industry.
Adequate involvement of whole family, helping it to accept the handicap and to learn how to cope with it.
Educational psychologist has important advisory and treatment role.
Need close cooperation between family, social, educational and medical agencies.

FURTHER READING

DHSS (1971) *Better Service for the Mentally Handicapped*. London: HMSO.
Dutton, G. (1975) *Mental Handicap*. London: Butterworths.
Heaton-Ward, W. A. (1977) *Left Behind*. London: MacDonald & Evans.
Mackay, R. I. (1976) *Mental Handicap in Child Health Practice*. London: Butterworths.
National Development Group for the Mentally Handicapped. Series of pamphlets obtainable from Room C412, Alexander Fleming House, Elephant and Castle, London SE1 6BY.
Series of articles by Kushlick, Nuttler, Corbett and Rutter in *Brit. J. Hosp. Med.*, August 1972.

The Mental Health Act 1983: some important issues

TERMINOLOGY

Mental handicap is only relevant if the clinical state fulfils the criteria of mental impairment, defined as a state of arrested or incomplete development of mind, which includes significant impairment of intelligence and social functioning and is associated with abnormally aggressive or seriously irresponsible conduct. The age limit for admission of patients with mental impairment is removed and replaced by a 'treatability' requirement (as in psychopathy below).

The term 'psychopathic disorder' is retained, but the age limit for detention of non-offenders for treatment has been abolished. Instead, at admission and renewal of detention there should be (as in the case of mental impairment) a criterion added that treatment is 'likely to alleviate or prevent a deterioration' of the patient's condition. A patient cannot be detained by reason only of promiscuity or other immoral conduct, nor by reason of sexual deviancy or dependence on drugs or alcohol.

COMPULSORY ADMISSION PROCEDURES

SECTION 2

Hospital admission for assessment (or for assessment followed by medical treatment).
Duration 28 days.
Application by nearest relative or approved social worker, either of whom must have seen the patient within 14 days of the application.
Medical recommendation: a) registered medical practitioner
                                  b) recognised specialist in mental illness
These doctors should have examined the patient together or separately, in the latter case not more than 7 days should have elapsed between the two examinations.

Patient has the right to appeal to a review tribunal within 14 days of admission to hospital.

SECTION 4

Hospital admission for assessment in emergency (when only one doctor is available and the degree of urgency does not permit delay for a second opinion).
Duration 72 hours from time of admission
Application by nearest relative or approved social worker, either of whom must have seen the patient within the previous 24 hours.
Medical recommendation. Registered medical practitioner (if possible one who previously knew the patient, preferably the family doctor). The patient must be admitted within 24 hours of the examination (or of the application if made earlier).

SECTION 136

Removal by police officer to place of safety of persons who appear to be mentally disordered in a place to which the public have access, if in immediate need of care or control.

SECTION 3

Admission for treatment. The specific form of mental disorder must be specified, and it must be such that hospital admission is the only appropriate method of management.
   Grounds for application under Section 3 are
a) that the patient is suffering from mental disorder, severe mental impairment, psychopathic disorder or mental impairment, being a disorder of a nature or degree which makes it appropriate for him to receive medical treatment in hospital, and
b) in the case of psychopathic disorder or mental impairment, that such a treatment is likely to alleviate or prevent a deterioration of his condition, and
c) that it is necessary for the health and safety of the patient or for the protection of other persons that he should receive such treatment and that it cannot be provided unless he is detained under this section.
Duration. 6 months, renewable for six months, then one year at a time.
Application. Nearest relative or approved social worker.
Recommendation: registered medical practitioner with previous knowledge of patient as well as recognised specialist in mental illness.

SECTION 5(2)
Emergency detention of informal patient already receiving psychiatric care in hospital.
Duration 72 hours from the time when the report is furnished.
Application. The responsible medical officer (i.e. consultant psychiatrist in charge of the case.) A suitably qualified nominated

deputy may act in place of the RMO. Patient may also be detained by a senior nurse (defined in the Act) for up to 6 hours until doctor arrives.

CONSENT TO TREATMENT

Fully informed (valid) consent means that the patient must
a) have full freedom of choice to accept or reject the treatment and is competent to judge the issue
b) understand the nature, purpose and effects of it
c) be fully aware of possible alternatives and the prognosis without treatment.

It has always been held as axiomatic that where possible the consent of both patient and nearest relative should be obtained before commencing any form of treatment involving risk.

The rules must be particularly strict and rigorous when compulsorily-detained patients refuse treatment. The Butler Committee recommended that treatment other than nursing care should not be imposed on any patient without his consent if he is able to appreciate what is involved. Three important exceptions were suggested:
a) where it is necessary to save the patient's life
b) where (not being irreversible) it is necessary to prevent him from deteriorating
c) where (not being of a hazardous or irreversible character) treatment represents the minimum interference with the patient to prevent him from behaving violently, or otherwise being a danger to himself or others.

The Butler Committee considered that such criteria may also apply if the patient is unable to appreciate what is involved despite the help of an explanation in simple terms.

The Butler Committee drew a clear distinction between irreversible or hazardous treatment (that which entails immediate significant physical hazard or having unfavourable irreversible physical or psychological consequences) and other treatments.

The 1983 Mental Health Act also distinguishes two kinds of treatment. The first applies to all patients. The second applies to detained patients only.

1. Requires consent *as well as* mandatory concurring second opinion from a doctor (appointed by the Mental Health Act Commission) as well as two non-medical opinions; only the doctor is expected to give an opinion on the validity of the proposed treatment. This group of treatments concerns hazardous and controversial methods such as leucotomy, stipulated under the Act.

2. Requires consent *or* (if the patient is unwilling or unable to give consent) a second opinion. This must be given by another doctor who should consult a nurse and one other professional concerned with the patient's treatment. This group of treatments includes ECT and such medication and other treatments as may be

stipulated in the Act. It does not apply to use of medicines (provided these are not in the 'limited' category) during the first three months following the first administration of medicines for the mental disorder, provided of course this falls within a period of time during which a patient is liable to be detained.

URGENT TREATMENT

The above conditions 1 and 2 do not apply to any treatment:
a) which is immediately necessary to save the patient's life
or
b) which (not being irreversible) is immediately necessary to prevent a serious deterioration of his condition
or
c) which (not being irreversible or hazardous) is immediately necessary to alleviate serious suffering by the patient
or
d) which (not being irreversible or hazardous) is immediately necessary and represents the minimum interference necessary to prevent the patient from behaving violently or being a danger to himself or to others.

MENTAL HEALTH ACT COMMISSION

This is a multidisciplinary and independent body whose role is to exercise a general protective function in respect of detained patients. It will visit hospitals regularly and appoint doctors to give second opinions. It will also publish an annual report and have some responsibility for informal patients.

MENTAL HEALTH TRIBUNALS

Patients detained under Section 2 may appeal to a tribunal within the first 14 days. Those under Section 3 may appeal in the first six months and the second six months and then every year of detention.

FURTHER READING

Review of the Mental Health Act 1959 DHSS (1978) Cmnd 7320 London: HMSO
NAMH (1975) *A Human Condition: the Mental Health Act from 1959 to 1975.* National Association of Mental Health
Report of the Committee on Mentally Abnormal Offenders (The Butler Committee) 1975 London: HMSO
Mental Health Act 1983 HMSO

Forensic psychiatry

GUILT AND INSANITY

The McNaghton rules
The accused shall only be regarded as insane to the point of
escaping responsibility for his criminal act if he was labouring
under such a deficit of reason, from disease of the mind, as not to
know the nature and quality of the act, or if he did know it, that
what he was doing was wrong.

These are extremely narrow, and strictly would only apply to
severely subnormals or delirium states. They reject notion of
irresistible or delusional impulses and are based on an intellectual
test of responsibility.

Interpretation has been loose and variable in recent years.

The Butler Committee recommended revising the special verdict
'not guilty by reason of insanity' to 'not guilty on evidence of
mental disorder'.
A. Evidence is given of mental disorder within the meaning of the
   Mental Health Act, negating a state of mind required for the
   offence (intention, foresight or knowledge).
B. Evidence is given of severe mental illness or severe
   subnormality. The relevant criteria of 'severe' are:
   1. Lasting impairment of intellectual function (memory,
      orientation, comprehension, learning capacity).
   2. Lasting alteration of mood of such a degree as to give rise to
      delusional appraisal of situation, or lack of appraisal.
   3. Delusional beliefs (persecutory, jealous, grandiose).
   4. Abnormal perceptions with delusional misinterpretation.
   5. Disordered thinking which prevents reasonable appraisal of
      situation or communication with others.
Butler Committee recommended discarding the criterion that
there was knowledge of wrongful nature of act. Home Office
Committee currently reviewing this.

FITNESS FOR TRIAL

If it is demonstrated that an accused person is insane and too mentally disturbed to be tried, he may be found 'unfit to plead' (or under disability).

Criteria of fitness to plead
Must be able to understand:
— the nature of the charge against him.
— the consequences of his plea of 'guilty' or 'not guilty'.
Must be able to:
— follow court procedure.
— instruct his defence counsel.
— object to the choice of individual jurors.

DIMINISHED RESPONSIBILITY

Introduced in the 1957 Homicide Act. Provides that a conviction of murder will be reduced to one of manslaughter if at the time of the act the accused was suffering from such an abnormality of mind as to substantially impair his mental responsibility for the act.

It thereby allows the sentence (for manslaughter) to be entirely at the discretion of the court.

PSYCHOPATHIC DISORDER

Definition
Scott abstracted 4 common factors in definition:
a) Exclusion of subnormality or psychosis.
b) Long standing duration.
c) Behavioural disorder: aggressive or irresponsible.
d) Society feels impelled to do something about it.

Under the 1983 Mental Health Act compulsory admission of psychopathic disorder for treatment must include the criterion that treatment is likely to alleviate or prevent a deterioration of the condition.

Prichard (1835): concept of moral as opposed to intellectual insanity.

Causes
47XYY genotype in high proportion of psychopathic offenders: tallness, immaturity of personality but no invariable association with low IQ. Hypogonadism. Probably only a few XYY individuals become persistently antisocial.

Immature slow wave pattern in EEG in up to 48% but interpretation requires caution (Hill).

Early parental deprivation and/or rejection stressed by some.
May be no cultural background of criminality.

Developmental environmental influence probably outweigh genetic.

Psychological immaturity probably an important factor.

Impaired early social learning causes vulnerability to later stresses and development of deviant social pathology.

Clinical features
Basic disorder is defective awareness of social behaviour.
Henderson suggested three types:
— predominantly aggressive.
— inadequate.
— creative.

Treatment
Conventional psychiatric inpatient unit of limited value. The Henderson Hospital therapeutic community (Maxwell Jones, Whiteley): recreates basic social learning situation, permissive, communal sharing of tasks and responsibilities, democratic decision-making, confrontation over 'here and now'. Some improvement in 41% at 1 year in creative psychopaths with some psychological maturity. Relatively ineffective in impulsive or aggressive psychopathy.
Not commonly used:
        Prison transfer to mental hospital
        residence in mental hospital as condition of probation
Treatment facilities grossly inadequate
Impulsive/aggressive type requires controlled setting as in prison
Inadequates require supportive regimes with benign authoritative direction
Creative type may respond to therapeutic community.

Natural history
Most destructive in early adult life.
Later become less antisocial though may remain so in family life.
High incidence of death by violence or suicide.

FURTHER READING

Briscoe, O. (1975) Assessment of intent: an approach to the preparation of court reports. *Brit. J. Psychiat.*, **127**, 461–465.

DHSS/Home Office (1975) *Report of the Committee on Mentally Abnormal Offenders*. London: HMSO.

Gunn, J. (1977) Criminal behaviour and mental disorder. *Brit. J. Psychiat.*, **130**, 317–329.

Pitcher, D. R. (1971) The XYY syndrome. *Brit. J. Hosp. Med.*, March, 379–393.

Whiteley, J. S. (1970) The psychopath and his treatment. *Brit. J. Hosp. Med.*, Feb., 263–270.

Treatments

A. PSYCHOTHERAPY

INDIVIDUAL SUPPORTIVE

Indications

Useful in two groups of patient:
1. Those experiencing stressful circumstances.
2. Those with chronic psychological problems or mental illness.

Aims:
— to help them to achieve best adaptation possible
— to reinforce existing personality structure and defence
— mechanisms.

Does not aim to achieve any radical change in personality or defence mechanisms.

Technique

Therapist adopts role of benevolent professional, fostering trust and positive expectations.

Permits patient to relinquish all or some of his self-reliance.

Dependent role sanctioned: patient need not feel shame or embarrassment.

Include in strategies:
— explanation
— encouragement, reassurance
— permission for catharsis
— environmental manipulation.

Basic rules:
Listen and say little. Avoid glib reassurance.
Do not interrogate. Encourage patient to be at ease.
Be empathic, accept patient non-judgementally.
Do not pronounce on general matters.
Avoid authoritative directions over what patient should do.
Avoid facile interpretations of behaviour and motives.
Keep own attitudes to oneself.
Do not over-identify with the patient (leads to excessive anxiety in therapist and impaired judgement).

Define aims clearly and the nature of help offered.
Set clear mutually agreed goals, frequency and duration of treatment.
Review progress regularly.
Respect confidentiality and avoid gossip.

Development of excessive dependency
The main complication. Liable to occur when therapist dominates and permits the patient too much passivity, fails to set mutually agreed goals from the start, or to review progress of therapy regularly.

FURTHER READING

Bloch, S. (1977) Supportive psychotherapy. *Brit. J. Hosp. Med.*, **18**, No. 1. July, 63–69.

FORMAL INDIVIDUAL PSYCHOTHERAPY: NON-DIRECTIVE (EVOCATIVE) PRINCIPLES

More intensive than supportive type, aims to achieve enduring personality change through a systematic scrutiny of the patient's past and present psychological life.
Promotes insight and encourages patient to discover answers himself.
Recollection and recounting of issues, feelings, situations.

Therapist interventions
Enquiry. Asking questions to elaborate patient's account.
Clarification. Pointing out and linking events so that patient is helped to understand repeated patterns in his feeling and thinking.
Explanation, interpretation. Offered as hypotheses for discussion. The precise content depends on theoretical model to be used. Occasionally used for the primary purpose of evoking emotional response (prokaleptic) rather than based on content validity.
Guidance of discussion. Ensure that emotionally painful but relevant topics are dealt with adequately rather than avoided.
Confrontation. Concerning inconsistencies, evasions and other defence mechanisms.

Therapist attitudes
Basic approach as for supportive therapy. In some variants, such as client-centred therapy, expression of therapist's own feelings is encouraged, together with 'genuineness, acceptance of patient with unconditional positive regard and accurate empathic understanding'.

FORMAL INDIVIDUAL PSYCHOTHERAPY: PSYCHOANALYTIC

A specialised form of non-directive (evocative) approach.

Freudian model

Therapist maintains a position of anonymity.

Techniques of free association: 5 daily sessions per week, each lasting 50 minutes.

Analyst interventions confined to elucidation of material, interpretation, confrontation, and reconstruction.

Analysand invests therapist with thoughts and feelings which originate from early experience. This is called the transference.

'Acting out' occurs when the transference affects behaviour outside the treatment situation.

Early interpretation requires a period of 'working through'.

Analysis of transference is central part of therapy.

Specific characteristics of a patient's transference reflect his psychopathology and 'transference neurosis' develops when earlier neurotic components dominate his feelings towards the analyst.

Repressed material is thereby repeated in the present, though its relationship to earlier experience is not recollected: it is an illusory apperception.

Transference may include element of positive regard and emotional attachment, or hostility and rejection.

Patient-therapist interaction may also reflect other processes: e.g. habitual attitudes, personality traits and behavioural styles which are not specially a matter of transference.

Resistance leads to suppression of unacceptable mental contents, avoidance of topics in association, and distortion of unconscious impulses which appear in disguise: therapy includes analysis of resistances.

FURTHER READING

Brown, J. A. C. (1961) *Freud and the Post Freudians*. Harmondsworth: Penguin.

Sandler, J., Dare, C. & Holder, A. A series of ten articles in the *British Journal of Psychiatry* between May 1970 and January 1971 outlines basic psychoanalytic concepts and their clinical application.

Further references to psychoanalytic and other approaches to psychotherapy may be found in the following very useful reports, published by Study Group of the Society of Clinical Psychiatrists:

A bibliography in Dynamic, Family and Social Psychiatry. (Chairman, John Birtchnell.)

The Place of Dynamic Psychiatry in Medicine. (Chairman, Heinz Wolff.)

CONJOINT PSYCHOTHERAPY FOR MARITAL PROBLEMS

50% of marriages encounter early adjustment problems.
10% of married couples experience sufficient difficulty to
contemplate or actually experience separation.
Most marital problems arise in first 2-3 years of marriage.
Divorce most frequent 6-7 years after marriage, and is
particularly common when one or both partners married before
18 years of age.
Divorce Reform Act, 1969. Formulated grounds for divorce in
terms of irretrievable marital breakdown.
   The traditional marital offences (desertion, adultery, cruelty,
incurable unsoundness of mind) are now mere components of
more general evidence of breakdown, and their collusional
manufacture is no longer necessary.

Fundamentals of conjoint therapy
Ideally:
   — adequate motivation in both partners, with a genuine wish
      to improve the relationship and to continue with it, and a
      willingness to accept the need for personal change where
      necessary.
   — neither partner is psychotic or so aggressive as to
      overwhelm the other in discussion.
   — each must be able to represent own views but be prepared
      to see other partner's too and compromise where
      necessary.
   — clear aims must be formulated and agreed by all concerned.
Therapist aims to:
   — facilitate communication.
   — avoid siding with one or other.
   — avoid directing and advising.
   — obey the rules of supportive psychotherapy.
   — resolve conflict rather than encourage a quarrel.
   — intervene to clarify, link aspects of behaviour or experience,
   — confront over inconsistencies, or interpret.
Preliminary individual therapy indicated:
   — when resistance to conjoint approach is severe.
   — when one partner is initially too disturbed.
   — when there is difficulty in sharing certain information.
   Conjoint therapy essential to resolve relationship problems and
avoids one partner being made into scapegoat. Can be useful in
treatment of married individuals even when problems are not
obviously related to marital relationship.
   Points which may be revealed by conjoint approach:
   — relative dominance of the partners.
   — cooperation or scapegoating.

- style of decision making (one-sided or mutually agreed).
- use of defence mechanisms.
- respective behaviour in the partners (over-controlling, acting-out, or over-inhibited and self-contained, degree of self-reflection or conscience-directed attitude).
- relative view of marriage boundaries (e.g. extra marital relations).

FURTHER READING

Crown, S. (1976) Marital breakdown: In *Recent Advances in Clinical Psychiatry–2*. Ed. Granville-Grossman, K., pp. 200–216. Edinburgh: Churchill Livingstone.
Dominian, J. (1968) *Marital Breakdown*. Harmondsworth: Penguin.

FAMILY PSYCHOTHERAPY

Based on the systems formed by individuals in families rather than focussed on individual psychopathology.

Indications
A family interview should be arranged when there is disorder of relationship, especially when the problem is not resolved by individual help.

Most useful when scapegoating and projective mechanisms marked.

Very disorganised families may need to be seen with other key individuals such as school staff.

Discussion of parental disharmony may act as reassurance for children, though it is inappropriate for them to be present when sexual problems of parents are dealt with.

Therapeutic processes
Variety of approaches. Therapist may direct, interreact or confront.
1. *Facilitation of communication*. Fundamental to all.
2. *Behavioural modification*. Learning theory principles.
3. *Psychoanalytic*. Deeper explorations needed when there is major resistance to change due to unconscious fantasies derived from childhood experiences. Transference already exists between marital partners, and therapist need not draw this on to himself. May be able to declare his own experiences (contrast individual therapy).
4. *General systems theory*. Based on principle that living systems are based on hierarchical sequence of supra and sub-systems which have boundaries between them. Within each there is a 'decider' mechanism. Resistance to change.

A family system needs a balance between open communication and sharing, versus separate autonomy.

Therapist may examine the way family resists change and tries to get him to collude in its psychopathology.

Outcome
Two studies suggest that short term crisis-orientated family therapy on out-patient basis is superior to conventional in-patient care (one quarter duration of disability, and time spent in hospital during subsequent 6 months may be halved). No significant difference in social and emotional functioning.

Spontaneous improvement occurs generally in family problems (66% in 2 years) but family therapy leads to more rapid resolution (86% in 1–3 weeks).

FURTHER READING
Skynner, A. C. R. (1976) Family and marital psychotherapy. *Brit. J. Hosp. Med.* March, 224–324.

GROUP PSYCHOTHERAPY

Five to eight patients meet with one or two therapists for one and a half hour session each week.

May be closed group: no new members admitted.
open group: members who leave are replaced by new ones.

Based on process of learning by sharing experiences and caring for others.

Selection of patients
Able to express ideas and feelings verbally.

Can withstand exposure to group process and make use of interpretations.

Applicable in a wide range of diagnostic categories, especially neurotic and psychosomatic conditions, but selection must take into account the needs of the particular group.

May be preferable to individual therapy in emotionally deprived individuals because regressive dependency on therapist is less likely.

Members should be matched approximately in educational level and social class, but mixed in sex.

Patients who are unsuitable
Paranoid or psychopathic personality.
Psychotics.
Narcissistic or schizoid with little interest in others.
Extreme rivalry for attention.
Marked sensitivity to distress of others.

Basic group processes

First phase
Anxiety, defensiveness, ambivalence toward leader.
Establishment of group culture.
Trust established by exchange of self-revelation.
Individual styles become clear.

Second phase
Each member reacts individually to the processes of sharing,
seeing the self in others, increased recognition of repressed
feelings, and free exploration of associations.

Common themes are competitiveness, fear of exposure, sexual
anxieties, dependency, autonomy.

Anti-therapeutic processes include scapegoating, development of
sub-group alliances, group defensiveness, pressure to confirm and
denial of differentiation.

Third phase
Before termination allow adequate working through of
implications. Some members may need further individual help.

Variants in technique

Bion
Traditional psychoanalytic: therapist confines remarks to
interpretations in terms of group transference to therapists.

Whitaker and Leiberman
Confrontation of individuals as well as the group.

Foulkes
Allows interaction between members unrelated to transference to
therapist.

Encounter groups
Emphasis on the present, discourages exploration of past,
avoidance of concepts such as the unconscious or ego defences.
Therapist declares own feelings readily. As in T groups and Gestalt
therapy, the leader is active, directing, with inspirational charisma.
May involve physical contact between members of group.

Evaluation of group therapy
Complex and difficult: repertory grid technique useful.

Truax: improvement in MMPI scores related to therapist empathy
and 'positive regard'.

Vigorous therapist involvement with confrontation and challenge
may lead to ill effects in members who have low self-esteem and
high expectations of treatment.

FURTHER READING

Marteau, L. (1976) Encounter and the new therapies. *Brit. J. Hosp. Med.*, March, 257–264.
Ryle, A. (1976) Group psychotherapy. *Brit. J. Hosp. Med.*, March, 239–248.
Walton, H. J. (1971) *Small Group Psychotherapy.* Harmondsworth: Penguin.

B. THE THERAPEUTIC COMMUNITY

Social therapy (Milieu Therapy) is the use of the milieu as a mode of treatment.

HISTORY

Tom Main: Northfield Military Hospital, later at the Cassell Hospital.
Maxwell Jones: Belmont Hospital, later at the Henderson Hospital.
Units later at Claybury, Fulbourne, Littlemore, Dingleton and Bethlem Hospitals.
Derivative approaches: Berne's Transactional Analysis, Perl's Gestalt Therapy.

CHARACTERISTIC FEATURES

Permissive, egalitarian, democratic, communalistic.
Total resource, both staff and patient, pooled in furtherance of therapy.
Patients are active agents of therapy and not passive recipients.
Small community, usually but not necessarily residential.
Reality confrontation, social analysis, face to face interchange.
Abolition of marks of differentiation such as titles, uniform.
Frequent total community meeting: regular daily and in crisis situation.
Constant adequate communication throughout the whole community.
Consensus decision making.

FURTHER READING

Clark, D. H. (1977) The therapeutic community. *Brit. J. Psychiat.*, **131**, 553–564.

C. BEHAVIOUR THERAPY

INDICATIONS

Adults
First choice in:
— phobic disorders, social anxiety, obsessive-compulsive rituals.

Useful in:
— sexual dysfunction e.g. impotence, frigidity
— sexual deviation e.g. exhibitionism
— obsessive thoughts
— habit disorders e.g. stammering, hair pulling, gambling
— appetite disorders e.g. obesity, anorexia nervosa
— social rehabilitation in chronic schizophrenia or organic defects.

Not of value:
— in acute schizophrenia, severe depression or hypomania
— whenever clear goals cannot be worked out.

Children
First choice in:
— nocturnal enuresis, phobias.
Useful in:
— educational rehabilitation of subnormal children or those with learning problems, conduct disorders.

TYPES

1. Reduce anxiety-linked behaviour (phobias, compulsive rituals) by exposure treatment such as desensitisation of flooding with self regulation, modelling.
2. Reduce appetitive behaviour (e.g. exhibitionism, obesity) by self regulation, satiation, aversion.
3. Develop new behaviour (e.g. learn social skills) by training, education programmes, modelling, shaping, self regulation, prompting, pacing, feeding, contracting, contingent reward.

PRINCIPLES

Clear delineation of treatment goals.
 Patient cooperation essential.
 Family involvement when psychopathology involves relatives.
 Treatment taken to relevant settings, e.g. home, restaurants, crowds.
 Inter-session home therapy by patient. Use of diary to rate anxiety, behaviour practice in anxiety-provoking situations.
 May need to use more than one therapeutic strategy.

EXPOSURE TECHNIQUE

Can produce significant improvement in phobias or compulsions
 Useful in social deficit and sexual dysfunction.
 Desensitisation in fantasy more rapid than with dynamic psychotherapy, though long term outcome similar.

Exposure *in vivo* for obsessive compulsive behaviour more effective than relaxation therapy and benefit still marked at 2 years (Marks 1976).

Techniques
Desensitisation. In fantasy only or *in vivo* by real life exposure to phobic situation. *In vivo* probably more effective. Graded hierarchy may not be essential.
Implosion. Exposure to maximal phobic situation until anxiety falls and feel better, either in fantasy or in real life situation.
Modelling. Demonstration of anxiety-provoking behaviour by therapist or relative.
Cognitive rehearsal and self regulation. Preparatory and concomitant reassurance, and techniques of self control of anxiety.
Response prevention. In compulsive rituals.

Theoretical basis
Based on principle that given enough contact with the provoking situation, the phobic or obsessive person ceases to respond with avoidance, distress or rituals. Patients rarely become sensitised to a situation through exposure. Paradox that exposure to trauma sometimes produces phobias and for others is curative.

Some advocate anxiety reduction as essential in therapy (Wolpe), others maintain it is irrelevant (Mark). Implosion implies that maximal anxiety is required during exposure for improvement to occur.

Deliberate provocation of anxiety (more than inherent in exposure) is not more effective.

Long therapeutic sessions (2 hours) better than several shorter ones probably because it allows time for development of self regulatory strategies.

A small minority of phobic panics do not respond to exposure: some helped by antidepressants or abreaction (when fear irrelevant to phobic situation or anger present).

AVERSION TECHNIQUES

Used less often. Elimination of maladaptive response is of value only if replaced by more adaptive one.

The aversive stimulus is presented at the same time as the stimulus that elicits the undesired behaviour and leads to a conditioned anxiety response. Little empirical evidence for this.

Punishment training requires presentation of aversion stimulus contingent upon actual performance of undesired response.

'Covert sensitisation'. Training in imagining of traumatic consequences of problem behaviour as well as imagining the behaviour itself.

TOKEN ECONOMIES

Increase in contingency reinforced behaviour in psychiatric in-patients (see Chesser review).

    Problem of implementation:

        rapid turn-over of ward staff

        non contingent reinforcement

        maintaining effect after leaving token economy

        enlisting patient's motivation.

CRITICAL EVALUATION OF BEHAVIOUR THERAPY

(American Psychiatric Association, Shapiro)

1. Based on experimental psychology. Caution in extending this to clinical situation.
2. Objective description and quantification of changes. May be unduly restricted to target symptoms.
3. Applicable to both psychological and organic illness. Need extreme caution in this approach to organic disease.
4. May help when psychotherapy has failed. Beware of placebo effect in evaluation.
5. Outcome evaluation used routinely. Rigorous criteria necessary here.
6. Experimental/control designs often used. True control can be difficult to define and obtain.
7. Claimed to be effective in many disorders: caution that claims do not outstrip the evidence. Behaviour therapy is a complex intervention and should not be over simplified.

FURTHER READING

Chesser, E. S. (1976) Behaviour therapy: recent trends and current practice. *Brit. J. Psychiat.*, **129**, 289–308.

Marks, I. M. (1976) The current status of behavioural psychotherapy: theory and practice. *Am. J. Psychiat.*, **133**, 253–261.

Shapiro, A. K. (1976) The behaviour therapies. Therapeutic break-through or latest fad? *Am. J. Psychiat.*, **133**, 154–159.

D. DRUGS

PHARMACOLOGY

Amines important in central nervous system transmission.

The anatomy of the 'amine system':

    Distribution of aminergic fibres demonstrated by fluorescent microscopy.

    Differentiation of neurones containing noradrenalin (NA) dopamine (DA) and serotonin (5-hydroxytryptamine 5HT)

    Amines are inactivated either by enzymatic action or by reuptake into nerve terminals.

5HT

Ho—[benzene ring fused with indole]—CH$_2$CH$_2$NH$_2$ Concentrated in midbrain raphe nuclei

N
H

DA

Ho—[benzene ring]—CH$_2$CH$_2$NH$_2$ Concentrated in substantia nigra, striatum,
Ho—   pituitary axis, arcuate nucleus of hypothalamus,
                                       limbic system

NA

Ho—[benzene ring]—CH(OH)CH$_2$NH$_2$
Ho—   Clustered in brain stem near fourth ventricle

PSYCHOTROPIC DRUGS

Those which act upon psychic functions, behaviour or experience.

Neuroleptics (antipsychotics, atarectics, major tranquillisers)

Phenothazines. Side chain — Dimethyl amino propyl (e.g.
                                chlorpromazine)
                   — piperazine (e.g. trifluoperazine)

Thioxanthenes (e.g. flupenthixol)

Butyrophenones (e.g. haloperidol)

May exert effects by inhibiting dopaminergic transmission through
receptor blockade (note extrapyramidal side effects, experimental
block of behavioural effects of stimulating nigrostrial pathway
which contains dopamine, and reduction of evoked potentials in
reticular formation from peripheral stimulation).

Side effects

Drowsiness, dry mouth, lactation in non-pregnant women, postural
hypotension, Parkinsonian syndrome, agranulocytosis, obstructive
(cholestatic) jaundice, photosensitivity, acute dystonic reaction,
(antidote benztropine 1–2 mg i.v.). Tardive dyskinesia (facial
involuntary movements) may be due to drug-induced
dopamine-receptor supersensitivity, a late complication of chronic
medication, especially high dosage and in older patients.

Anxiolytic sedatives (minor tranquillisers)
Reduce pathological anxiety, tension and agitation, but no therapeutic effect on disturbed cognitive or perceptual aspects of psychosis. Cause little autonomic or extra-pyramidal side effects.

Benzodiazepines may lead to tolerance, physical dependence and withdrawal symptoms. In some (e.g. diazepam) the long half life may mean that withdrawal symptoms can occur up to a week after drug stopped. Can cause drowsiness, ataxia and occasionally (paradoxically) aggression.

Antidepressants
Affective illness may be due to failure in aminergic transmission. Antihypertensive drugs reserpine and α methyldopa (which deplete the central nervous system of catecholamine derivatives) also may cause severe depression. It is not clear whether NA or 5HT involved.

Tricyclics
May act by blocking re-uptake process across the neuronal membrane through competition for NA receptors.

Side effects: dry mouth, urinary retention and constipation (anticholinergic effects), postural hypotension, drowsiness, blood dyscrasias, jaundice(rare), ECG changes (flat T waves), sudden death in patients with prexisting heart disease, glaucoma.
Monoamine oxidase inhibitors (MAOIs) lead to striking rise in levels of 5HT and DA in brains of experimental animals. Should not be used at same time as drugs that block re-uptake of NA (e.g. amphetamine) or tyramine-containing foods (see p. 49) which release NA from sympathetic nerve terminals and may cause hypertensive crisis when taken with MAOIs.
   MAOIs may also potentiate hypoglycaemia (caution in diabetics) and potentiate effects of morphine-like analgesics and anaesthetics (due to inhibition of hepatic enzymatic breakdown).

L tryptophan. May be useful in treatment of depression when used in conjunction with MAOIs (rationale: its metabolite 5-hydroxyindole acetic acid levels low in CSF of depressed patients. Tryptophan is a precursor of 5-HT).

Lithium carbonate
Used as prophylactic in mania. Also of value in treating acute mania.

Prior to use check: cardiovascular, renal, hepatic and thyroid functions.

Side effects: tremor, ataxia, abdominal distension, constipation, vomiting, diarrhoea (when these develop, stop drug and check serum levels), mild non-toxic goitre, hypothyroidism (block of thyrotropic hormone), and diabetes insipidus. Fatal delirium, coma in overdose: slow excretion hinders treatment (more than 95% via kidneys, hence beware of renal impairment). Nephrotoxicity also possible.

FURTHER READING

Lader, M. (1980) *Introduction to Psychopharmacology.* Upjohn Scope.

E. ELECTROCONVULSIVE THERAPY (ECT)

HISTORY

Early observation by mental hospital physicians: patients tended to lose their symptoms when they had a spontaneous convulsion.
   Epilepsy and schizophrenia rarely concurrent in the same patient.
   Von Meduna 1935: induced fits using i.m. camphor in oil.
   Cerletto and Bini 1933: electroshock first used.

PROBLEMS OF EVALUATION

Comparison of evaluative studies difficult because of heterogeneous patient groups and variation in diagnostic practice, failure to differentiate acute from chronic illness. Fully 'blind' control studies are rare (i.e. control involves giving anaesthesia without ECT) and ethically questionable.
   As yet only equivocal evidence that convulsion (as opposed to anaesthetic plus elaborate procedure) is essential therapeutic component.

EFFECTIVENESS

Depressive illness
R. C. Psychiatrists Memorandum concluded that there is substantial and incontrovertible evidence that ECT is effective in severe depressive illness.
   The most comprehensive studies suggest it is at least as effective as antidepressant medication, and quicker in action.
   'Endogenous' type symptoms respond most readily but indication for ECT should be on basis of severity of depression and need for rapid response.
   Status of unilateral versus bilateral ECT uncertain.

Two major early trials (random allocation of patients but not double blind)

Greenblatt et al., 1964. Multicentre, 281 depressed patients, 8-week trial period. Overall marked improvement with ECT 76%; imipramine 49%; phenelzine 50%; isocarboxazid 28%; placebo 46%. (ECT significantly better than any other at 1% level significance.)

   M.R.C. 1965. 269 patients with depressive illness as primary diagnosis. At 4 weeks nil or only slight symptoms: ECT 71%; Imipramine 52%; Phenelzine 30%; Placebo 39%. At 4 weeks only female patients responded better to ECT than to imipramine and at 6 months the responses in the ECT and Imipramine group were identical.

   Some smaller studies have shown only minimal or no difference in effectiveness of ECT and antidepressants.

Double blind trials: four recently carried out in Britain

Freeman et al 1978: Edinburgh. Bifrontal sinusoidal ECT twice weekly, compared with two simulated treatments in first week followed by real treatment. At end of first week the group receiving real ECT showed significantly greater improvement (on observer rating and one of two self report ratings) than control group. Subsequently the simulated treatment group required greater number of ECT applications.

Lambourne & Gill 1978: Southampton. Comparison of real and simulated brief pulse unilateral ECT applied ×3 weekly for 2 weeks. Both groups improved, and the only significant advantage of real ECT was in relief of hypochondriacal symptoms (although even this was regarded as fortuitous).

West 1981: Sutton. Real compared with simulated ECT, twice weekly, bifrontal sinusoidal. Striking improvement with real ECT after 1 week, but no change in control group. Trial allowed patients not showing improvement after six treatments to be transferred to other group, and subsequently it was found that this option had been chosen in ten of the eleven patients who had started on simulated ECT, but in none who had commenced with real ECT. The ten 'switched' patients improved as soon as they received real ECT.

Johnstone et al, 1980: Northwick Park. Real and simulated ECT compared, total of eight applications twice weekly, bifrontal sinusoidal. Both groups improved steadily during treatment. At end of 4 weeks only modest advantage of real ECT, restricted to patients with delusions. At 1 and 6 months no significant differences between the two groups.

Possible Explanation for Different Findings in these Studies
Unilateral ECT used in Southampton study may be relatively
ineffective form of treatment, and it may also have been difficult to
be sure that bilateral convulsion occurred. Variation in patient
selection may also have been important. Only 22% of Northwick
Park patients had received ECT previously (compared with 55–66%
in other studies) and they comprised 64% of all psychiatric
in-patients admitted for treatment of depression. This very high
proportion may explain why so many of the simulated treatment
group recovered so quickly in this study.
   Long term outcome data, comparable to Northwick Park data,
required in all studies if comparison is to be useful.

Mania and hypomania
No satisfactory controlled studies. Some retrospective studies
suggest that ECT leads to quicker and more complete recovery. The
important question is whether ECT is better than drugs.

Schizophrenia
Recent study of Taylor & Fleminger (1980). Acute schizophrenia not
responding to drugs randomly allocated to real or simulated ECT
8–12 applications. Significantly greater initial improvement with
real ECT, but no difference at 16 weeks. It remains possible that
longer course might have more lasting effect.
   Generally agreed that ECT is of little value in chronic
schizophrenia.

Unilateral versus bilateral ECT
Royal College Psychiatrists Memorandum concludes that it is
uncertain whether unilateral or bilateral ECT is more effective in
depression. (In 29 studies, unilateral less effective in 13, identical in
14, more effective in 2.)
   D'Elia and Raotmo suggest that non-dominant unilateral ECT has
the same antidepressant effect as bilateral but causes fewer side
effects such as memory impairment.
   Some clinical impressions suggest that bilateral ECT acts more
quickly in severe depression and few applications needed, but
others disagree.

MORTALITY OF ECT

Surveys estimate 3–9 deaths per 100 000 ECT applications.
(Compare mortality dental OP anaesthesia 0.3 per 100 000.)
   Before ECT introduced, mortality in severe depressives 15% in 10
year period.
   Recent 3 year follow up of 519 depressed patients showed much
lower mortality in those who had received ECT.

Cholinergic effects of muscle relaxants may lead to serious cardiac dysrhythmias, and routine use of atropine to block this is imperative in ECT.

MORBIDITY DUE TO ECT

Immediate:
- — headaches and temporary confusion.
- — memory loss for recent events, diminishes rapidly after the final application but may increase with the number used.

Long term:
- — no objectively demonstrated memory impairment.
- — patients who have received bilateral ECT, subjectively rate memory as impaired 6–9 months later more frequently than do those who received unilateral ECT.

May be minor permanent loss of memory limited to events shortly before the time of treatment: effect increases with number and frequency of treatments and more likely with bilateral rather than unilateral ECT. Not likely to occur if treatment frequency is two or less per week.

'Kindling' phenomenon: sporadic grand mal fits for first time in the weeks or months after ECT rare, and do not persist over more than one year.

ECT induces extensive EEG changes: bilateral paroxysmal delta waves subside rapidly after treatment completed, and EEG usually returns to normal within three months.

TECHNIQUE OF ADMINISTRATION

Preparation
Full physical examination imperative.
Any significant organic disease discussed with general physician, anaesthetist.
Particular caution with cardio vascular disease (especially valvular).
Contra indications: recent cardiac infarction, severe pulmonary disease.
Ensure: availability of all medical/nursing notes at time of treatment.
- — resuscitatory equipment.
- — nursing staff.
- — overnight fasting.

Treatment
Anaesthetic given by anaesthetist (atropine, thiopentone, scoline).
Beware of prolonged paralysis due to pseudocholinesterase deficiency.
Oxygenate well before ECT given, and afterwards until normal breathing is re-established.

Avoid sub convulsions: cause headache and anxiety.
Use least possible amount of current (memory disorder proportional to the amount used).
Machine should have choice of wave form and automatic timing.
If no convulsion, repeat application up to maximum of 3.
Electrodes placed over fronto temporal areas in bilateral treatment (some claim that memory is less impaired if placed over frontal or occipital areas).
In unilateral treatment electrodes placed on mastoid and temporal regions of same side.
   After convulsion:
      — patient is oxygenated with airway *in situ.*
      — patient remains under anaesthetist's supervision until spontaneous respiration returns and regains consciousness.
      — close nursing supervision in ECT room (watch for respiratory difficulties, cardiac arrest) and later in recovery room when reassurance and explanation important.
      — allow rest for about 1 hour.
   Usual number of treatments 6. Given regularly usually twice weekly.
   Little justification for daily application: probably increases memory disturbance.
   Monitor response regularly.
   Antidepressant drugs may prevent relapse after treatment stopped and reduce number of applications needed.
   A report to the Royal College of Psychiatrists recommends: a consultant should be responsible for each ECT clinic, teaching and training junior staff in the theory and practice of ECT, should be personally involved in the clinic and ensure adequate standards.
   Need to improve standard of ECT facilities. Each clinic should:
a) specify the type of stimulus to be used, placement of electrodes, procedure to be followed if first stimulus fails to produce a fit, and the way atropine is to be used.
b) keep a patient register (name, date of attendance, number of ECTs in present and past courses, complications).
c) keep a separate card index on each patient with details of treatment, anaesthetic, relaxant, electrode position, stimulus, effect.
d) ensure that full case notes are available, and that the anaesthetist is aware of the obligatory physical examination, current drug therapy and drug sensitivities.
e) ensure that both a written account of what ECT involves as well as verbal explanation is given to the patient and, where appropriate, to relatives.
f) use only up to date safe equipment: Ectron Constant Current apparatus and Series 4 machines (After 1979).
g) titrate length of treatment (number of applications) against clinical response.

MEDICO LEGAL ASPECTS

Fully informed written consent: both doctor and patient should sign to the effect that explanation has been given. Applies to both informal and detained patients. Single consent adequate for each course of treatment but patient may withdraw consent at any time.

Two doctors should be present when ECT given, one experienced in anaesthesia.

If patient unwilling to have ECT or unable to understand what is proposed, consultant reconsiders alternatives.

If ECT essential and considered safe, then a Treatment Order (Section 3) is needed to proceed and except in an emergency a written second medical opinion is required stating that although consent cannot be obtained, ECT is necessary in order to alleviate or prevent deterioration. Two other professionals concerned with the patient must also be consulted (one a nurse).

FURTHER READING

D'Elia, G., & Raotmo, H. (1975) Is unilateral ECT less effective than bilateral ECT? *Brit. J. Psychiat.*, **126**, 83–89.
Kendell, R. E. (1981) The present status of electroconvulsive therapy. *Brit. J. Psychiat.*, **139**, 265–284.
Pippard, J., & Ellam, L. (1981) Electroconvulsive treatment in Great Britain: a report to the College. *Brit. J. Psychiat.*, **139**, 563–569.
Royal College of Psychiatrists (1977) Memorandum on the use of ECT. *Brit. J. Psychiat.*, **131**, 261–272.

F. PSYCHOSURGERY

HISTORY

1936 Moniz. Division of frontal lobe white matter to quieten aggressive behaviour. Awarded Nobel Prize 1949.

1942 Freeman and Watts. Standard leucotomy extensively used until early 1950s. At least 10 000 performed in U.K. between 1942–1952. (66% chronic schizophrenia, 33% affective illness. Usually chronic illness with severe behaviour disorders prior to neuroleptic drug era.)

Imprecise, blind operation, serious complications common (apathy, flat affect, euphoria, disinhibition, aggression, intellectual impairment, incontinence, epilepsy, metabolic disorders).

Early 1950s advent of neuroleptic drugs, and leucotomy virtually superceded.

Subsequently, limits of drug therapy clear. Renewed interest in leucotomy (restricted, involving stereotaxis which permits precision in size and site of lesion).

Lesions used include cold, heat, cutting or electrical stimulation.

NEUROANATOMY AND NEUROPHYSIOLOGY

Profound autonomic and emotional changes induced by artificial stimulation of limbic system and amygdala.

Frontal lobe monitors and modulates limbic mechanisms.

Fronto limbic connections (4 main pathways):
  — dorsal convexity via cingulate gyrus to hippocampus
  — dorsal convexity to hypothalamus, mesencephalon
  — orbital surface to septum
  — orbital surface to hypothalamus.

Psychosurgery aims at:
  — fronto limbic connections and where these are concentrated, viz, in the lower medial quadrant and posterior orbital area of the frontal lobes and the cingulate gyrus
  — limbic circuits
  — the limbic core.

EFFECTIVENESS AND COMPLICATIONS

Lesions of anterior cingulate gyrus

Electrical stimulation under local anaesthesia and stereotactic techniques used to aid target location (Kelly).

Particularly effective in obsessional neurosis, especially when anxiety and depression prominent. Less effective in depression alone.

Lesions of ventromedial frontal lobe

These include bifrontal subcaudate tractotomy using Yttrium 90 isotope implant (Knight), orbital undercutting or bimedial operations (Schurr).

Particularly useful in severe depression, agitation and tension. Recovered or much improved: 60% depressives, 40–60% anxiety states, 50% obsessionals.

No affective blunting, reduced incidence of suicide attempts.

Lesions of amygdala or temporal lobes

Temporal lobectomy in:
  — epileptics with aggressive outbursts (Turner).
  — drug resistant epilepsy, when focal disease confined to non dominant temporal lobe or the anterior 5–6 cm of the dominant lobe. Abolish fits in 50% when underlying lesions is mesial temporal sclerosis, less effective in other disorders.

INDICATIONS FOR PSYCHOSURGERY

Advised by its exponents: in obsessionals, depression and anxiety states when other therapy has failed and illness relentless, disabling, becoming chronic.

When good previous personality and absence of psychopathy. Free from organic brain and cerebrovascular disease.

Based on assumption that gross abnormality of limbic function may lead to intractible depressive, anxiety or obsessional neurosis.

Aims to restore neurophysiological balance without altering personality.

Not now used in schizophrenia unless above symptoms predominate.

Not acceptable as a way of controlling antisocial behaviour unless this is complication of relevant psychiatric disorder (e.g. temporal lobe epilepsy).

The Mental Health Act 1983 requires that in all cases of proposed leucotomy there should be concurring second medical and two non-medical written recommendations, as well as fully-informed consent.

When social/interpersonal factors are relevant to the illness, psychosurgery should not be undertaken until these have been fully treated and are clearly intractible. Insufficient attention to this point in recent literature.

REHABILITATION

Careful nursing supervision: monitor mood swings and suicide risk, retraining to avoid return of obsessional habits and to establish new routines.

FURTHER READING

Bridges, P. K. & Bartlett, J. R. (1977) Psychosurgery, yesterday and today. *Brit. J. Psychiat.*, **131**, 249–260.
Kelly, D. (1976) Neurosurgical treatment of psychiatric disorders. In *Recent Advances in Clinical Psychiatry – 2*. Ed. Granville-Grossman, K. pp. 227–261. Edinburgh: Churchill Livingstone.
Schurr. P. H. (1973) Psychosurgery. *Brit. J. Hosp. Med.*, July, 53–59.

Special topics

A. SUICIDE

DEFINITION

WHO (1968): a suicidal act with fatal outcome.
Beck (1976): a wilful self inflicted life threatening act which has resulted in death.

STATISTICS

Assessment of intent difficult:
— ambivalent motivation frequent.
— often has to be inferred in absence of explicit evidence.
International comparison difficult: variation in categorisation, which may be carried out either by medical or legal personnel.

In some countries proof of intent (e.g. a note) is required before a death is classed as suicide. Otherwise open verdict recorded.

Official statistics may under-estimate incidence of suicide: in Dublin perusal of psychiatric records suggests true incidence 4 × official rate (McCarthy & Walsh).

If open verdicts are mainly concealed suicides, then official statistics are 22% too low.

High rank-consistency in suicide rates of various countries and of London Boroughs over prolonged period of time, irrespective of the individual coroner involved.

In the U.K. and U.S.A. suicide accounts for 1% of all deaths.

AGE, SEX

Incidence increases with age.
More common in males than females in all age groups.
In England and Wales: suicide rate in 1978 was 8.2 per 100 000 persons over 15 years of age.
Compare rate of 15.1 per 100 000 in 1962.
During period 1901–1970: marked fall in rates for older males, increase in younger males and in females of all ages.

The fourth commonest cause of death in young adults.
1 in 800 000 age group 10–14 years.
Extremely rare in children under 10 years old.

URBAN/RURAL

Urban rates greater than in rural areas but in recent years the difference has been less marked.

MARITAL STATUS

Incidence greater in divorcees, widows, widowers, than in single or never married.

SEASON

Highest incidence in April, May, June in northern hemisphere; during period spring to mid summer in Australia.
Seasonal variation more marked in females.

SOCIAL CLASS

Highest in Class V (unskilled).
Moderate increase in Class I (professional) and IV (partly skilled).
Lower than expected in Class II and III (lower professionals and executives, skilled manual and non-manual).

ETHNIC AND RELIGIOUS GROUP

Rates previously low in black Americans, but recent increase in young black suicide to level of whites.
Relation to religious persuasion complex. Durkheim's finding of greater incidence in Protestants than Catholics not universally applicable today.

METHOD

In England and Wales since 1963: remarkable drop in number due to domestic gas, related to reduction of carbon monoxide content of town gas. About one third suicides due to this early 1960s, falling to near zero in 1972.
Increase in drug poisoning (67% female, 37% male) particularly due to antidepressants, tranquillisers and salicylates.
Fall in barbiturate poisoning, though this was still the cause of 27% of all suicides in 1973 in England and Wales.
Violent method more common in males.
Use of firearm much more common in U.S.A. than in U.K.

CORRELATES OF SUICIDE

Age over 40 years. Male more often than female.
Widowed, divorced, separated.
Immigrant.
Live alone, poor social contact and support.
Unemployed, retired.
Live in socially disorganised area.

Family history of affective disorder, suicide, alcoholism.
Previous history of affective disorder, alcoholism.
Previous suicide attempt.
Early in treatment for depression or soon after discharge from psychiatric hospital.
Addiction to alcohol, especially when significant complications present.
Incapacitating terminal illness in elderly.
Bereavement, separation, loss of job.

Personality: cyclothymic, sociopathic.
Mental illness:
   — severe depression
   — alcoholism, other addictions
   — early dementia
   — organic brain syndromes (epilepsy, head injury).
Symptoms:
   — depressed mood, persistent insomnia, loss of interests, hopelessness, self blame, agitation or retardation, social withdrawal, suicidal thoughts.
Attempted suicide:
   — precautions taken to prevent discovery, elaborate preparation, violent method or use of more lethal poison.

MANAGEMENT AND PREVENTION

Recognition of high risk groups
Suicide occurs in:
11 – 17% of severe (psychotic) depressions
7% of epileptics who also have organic brain syndromes
2% of schizophrenics
drug addicts at 50 × rate in general population
severe physical illness (a factor in 29% of suicides).
Note the danger of certain drugs which cause depression (reserpine, depot phenothiazines, barbiturates, contraceptives).

Psychotherapy
Recognition and support for individuals in crisis especially the severely depressed.
   May need hospital admission or regular supportive help.

Physical treatment

Recent study showed that 82% of suicides were receiving prescribed psychotropic drugs at time of death. (Barraclough et al., 1974).

Irregularities in their use included:
— failure to use antidepressants specifically for depressive illness
— use of too low doses
— continued for many months
— Excessive prescription of barbiturates and phenothiazines
— use of depot phenothiazines in non schizophrenic illnesses

ECT needed in severe depression when immediate suicide risk severe.

Community services

In U.S.A. Suicide Prevention Centres developed.

In U.K. Emphasis on voluntary agencies in collaboration with statutory services.

The Samaritans shown to attract high risk individuals.

Relative decline in suicide rate in towns where they operate (Bagley 1968) interpretation difficult because of many other potentially relevant social factors. Negative findings in more recent study (Jennings).

FURTHER READING

Barraclough, B. et al. (1974) A hundred cases of suicide: clinical aspects. *Brit. J. Psychiat.*, **125**, 355–373.

Jennings, C. (1978) Have the Samaritans led to a reduction in the suicide rate? *Psychol. Med.* **8**, 413–422.

Lancet (1978) Leading article: Suicide and the Samaritans. *Lancet* ii, 772.

Sainsbury, P. (1973) Suicide: opinion and fact. *Proc. Roy. Soc. Med.*, **66**, 579–587.

B. NON FATAL DELIBERATE SELF HARM (DSH)

(*parasuicide, attempted suicide*)

DEFINITION

A non fatal act in which an individual deliberately causes self injury or ingestion of a substance in excess of any prescribed or generally recommended therapeutic dose (Kreitman).

A deliberate non-fatal act, whether physical, drug overdosage or poisoning, done in the knowledge that it was potentially harmful, and in the case of drug overdosage, that the amount taken was excessive (Morgan).

Recent definitions attempt to avoid interpretation of whether conscious intent of self destruction was present, because this is difficult to detect reliably and many episodes are not associated with conscious ideas of suicide.

INCIDENCE

Since early 1960s increased progressively at 10% per annum in western countries.

Overall rates in 1972 (per 100,000)	Male	Female
Edinburgh	366	219
Oxford	354	170
Southampton	355	213
Bristol	307	157

METHOD

Drug overdosage in 93% (psychotropic drugs 49%, barbiturates 14%, salicylates 17%).

In London nearly 50% of episodes seen in hospital accident departments involve more than one drug.

78% use prescribed drugs (67% their own, 11% other persons).

Hypnotic overdose more common in older patients, tranquillisers in 20–34 year age group, and analgesics in young adults (79% of those age 15–19 years who resort to DSH).

Recent alcohol intake within preceding 6 hours in 50% male and 25–45% female DSH patients.

Self laceration:
  — in 5–10% of those attending hospital.
  — a few are males who are severely depressed and inflict single deep coarse incision near vital point.
  — majority are females with delicate, superficial and multiple incisions, less commonly associated with overt depression.

Repetition of DSH in 25% males and 23% females in year after episode.

CORRELATES

Marked difference in incidence according to living conditions: high in central disorganised urban areas, where overcrowding, lack of amenities are marked and high proportion of population unskilled. Also high in local authorities council housing estates. Low in middle class areas (professional, managerial, skilled artisan).

Important to recognise that ecological correlates may have only indirect significance: only 7% DSH patients themselves live in overcrowded conditions.

Early parental separation: 34% men, 26% women.
Previous criminal record: 30% men, 6% women.
Unemployment: 5 × expected rate.

64% some major precipitating event.
50% interpersonal upset.
Less commonly, anxiety over work or finance, illness, housing,
bereavement, antisocial behaviour.
25% no upset admitted.

45% do not have close friend, 35% feel personally isolated at all times.

Major psychotic illness	14% males	11% females
Chronic alcohol abuse	25%	7%
Alcohol intake within 6 hours	55%	25%
Reactive depression	39%	59%
Personality disorder	42%	22%
Organic psychosis	17%	6%

MOTIVATION AND CAUSES

	Male(%)	Female(%)
At the time of DSH wish to die	46	34
By the next day regret not dying	17	10
Evidence of serious intent to die	10	10

The majority are impulsive acts in relation to upsetting event which
precipitates depression in someone who is vulnerable, but only a
small minority mentally ill. Facilitated by recent intake of alcohol.
   Reasons given for the episode:
   — seek help
   — escape from situation
   — relief from state of mind
   — attempt to influence someone.
   Ordeal character: gamble between life and death
   Appeal or communicational effect: 18% are aware of one or more
similar episode in first degree relative.
   Self laceration may have obsessional-compulsive character in
some, or hysterical change in state of consciousness with
anaesthesia of mortified part. Can be a difficult problem in prisons
or other institutions in which freedom of movement limited.
Secondary gain may be important, often in impulsive aggressive
personality.
   Alcohol problems most marked in middle aged men and in those
living in city centres.
   Inappropriate prescription of psychotropic drugs also important.

COMPARISON BETWEEN SUICIDE AND NON FATAL DELIBERATE SELF HARM (DSH)

Suicide
Overall rates falling.

Rates increase with age.
Rare in children.
More common in males.
Drug poisoning most common cause but physical violence not infrequent.

DSH
Marked increase in rates since early 1960s
Rates fall as age increases.
Rare in children.
More common in females.
Massive preponderance of drug overdosage.
Only minority have conscious idea of suicide. 1% commit suicide in following year (10% in long term), only 10% are 'failed suicides'.

PREDICTION OF REPETITION

At 0.001 level
    Previous episode of DSH, psychiatric treatment or criminal record.
At 0.01 level   ╻
    Social Class IV or V, separated, episode not precipitated by upset, drug dependence, early separation (before 15 years) from mother.

ASSESSMENT AFTER DSH FOR HIGH RISK SUICIDE OR REPEAT NFDSH

Age and sex. Males age 35 years or older.
    Act of DSH. Severe, especially extensive laceration, precaution to avoid discovery, premeditated 24 hours or more, no obvious precipitating factors, conscious suicide intent.
    Preceding symptoms. Persistent depression, self blame, anger, resentment, impulsive behaviour, psychosis, serious alcohol or drug problem, serious physical discord, persistent somatic symptoms.
    Social. Recurrent crises, lack support, separated, live alone, in city centre.
    Personal. Suicide in first degree relative, separated from parents for six months or more before age 15 years, episode of DSH is previous three months, previous psychiatric treatment.
    Status after episode. Persistent depression, anger, resentment, uncooperative, continuing suicidal ideas, unresolved or worsening situation.

TREATMENT AND PREVENTION

The Hill Report in 1968 recommended that all cases of deliberate self harm should be referred to designated Treatment Centres in District General Hospitals and seen by psychiatrists.
Implementation of this advice has been very incomplete and considerable variation exists in the way these patients are treated.

It has been demonstrated that in certain circumstances, medical practitioners (other than psychiatrists), nurses and social workers can be as effective as psychiatrists in the initial psychosocial evaluation of patients admitted to hospital following DSH. Delegation of psychiatric responsibility should however only occur in a well organised scheme where prompt psychiatric advice is readily available and good communication exists between all staff involved, who also obtain adequate preliminary training in assessment of suicide and DSH risk.

Each service should establish a clearly laid down code of practice concerning the management of patients who have deliberately harmed themselves, specifying:
— who is to carry out assessment.
— inter-professional referral procedures, including prompt communication with general practitioners.
— arrangement for prompt transfer of certain patients to psychiatric units.
— after-care arrangements.
— collection of appropriate statistics for monitoring purposes.
— detailed arrangements for children and young people.

Even though 50–55% of cases are referred to psychiatric clinics, they show a high default rate.

No effective way of reducing repetition rate yet demonstrated, either using psychiatric or social work techniques.

'First ever' cases respond best.

Patients show variety of attitudes to help: 36% prefer G.P., 23% are recurrent psychiatric attenders, 41% do not readily seek help from anyone.

Psychotherapy often involves:
long term support setting limits
treatment of significant depression
use of conjoint situation

Primary prevention may be most fruitful approach (early intervention, provision of adequate support especially when psychotropic drugs prescribed for persons with life difficulties).

FURTHER READING

Hawton, K., & Catalan, J. (1982) *Attempted Suicide*. Oxford: Oxford University Press.
Kreitman, N. (Ed.) (1977) *Parasuicide*. Chichester: John Wiley.
Morgan, H. G. (1979) *Death Wishes?* Chichester: John Wiley.

C. MENTAL HEALTH SERVICES

PREVALENCE OF MENTAL DISORDER

National Morbidity Survey 1970–1971. Office of Population Census and Surveys.

Based on 53 general practices in England and Wales.
1 in 14 males ⎱ consult a general practitioner because
1 in 7 females ⎰ of mental illness per year.
Of these 12% referred to specialist services.

Anxiety state   20 male, 47 female ⎱
Depressive neurosis 15 male, 47 female ⎰ per 1000 attended G.P.
Affective psychosis 1 in 280.
Schizophrenic psychosis 1 in 300.

PATTERN OF PSYCHIATRIC SERVICES

Since 1950s progressive increase in emphasis on community based facilities as opposed to those in large psychiatric hospitals.
Uncertainty regarding the future role of mental hospitals.
Progressive fall in numbers of patients requiring long term hospital care.

THE HEALTH DISTRICT	Population approximately 250 000	
Mental Health Service Provision (Adults)	Beds per 100,000	Day places
Psychiatric units in district		
general hospital	50	65
Elderly severely mentally infirm	30–40	25–40
New long stay patients	31	
Peripheral day hospital		30
Local Authority Provision (Adults)		
Hostels in community	4–6	
Long stay accommodation	15–24	
Day centre		60

Increasing emphasis on voluntary agencies in providing comprehensive service.

The District General Hospital (DGH) Psychiatric Unit is intended as the centre of specialist psychiatric treatment for adults, including compulsorily detained patients.

The majority will be ambulant, stay for a few weeks only.

Rather more than half day places used by inpatients.

The Elderly Mentally Infirm (*EMI*) would be treated separately, or together with other psychiatric patients in DGH unit.

A few (ESMI) will need continuing care usually because of dementia: preferably in small community hospitals (2.5–3.0 per 1000 age 65+).

Joint assessment unit with geriatricians (e.g. 10–20 beds for this purpose in each health district).

As population gets older the required facilities for the elderly will increase considerably in the next few decades. The population in the year 2000 compared with the present will be: total: 104%; 64–75 years: 90%; 75 years and over: 128%.

Long term care of chronic mental illness
In 1971, of patients in mental illness hospital, 73% had been there more than one year, 41% more than ten years.

Excluding dementia, other forms of chronic mental illness still develop.

The new long stay patients who stay in hospital 1–3 years.
Sample evaluated by Mann and Cree.
One third need continuous medical/nursing supervision.
Remainder need sheltered environment in community.
0.17 per 1000 beds required in each health district.
Ideal placement uncertain. DGH units not most suitable. Hostel near hospital campus may be best.

Chronic Organic Brain Damage
Placements a problem especially when behaviour disorder complicates it.

Services for children
Continued expansion of hospital services a high priority.
Prime emphasis will need to be on early intervention in home, school, health centre and other community bases.
Close collaboration between many agencies required and involvement of whole families as well as other key personnel.

Services for adolescents
Evidence that psychiatric morbidity is higher than in adults, yet adolescents reluctant to seek help.
Special needs must be taken into account.
Informal walk-in clinics useful.
Voluntary agencies invaluable in providing this approach.

FUTURE OF THE MENTAL HOSPITAL

Aim at a period of transition rather than dissolution.
Emphasis increasingly towards day hospital and other community care.
The DGH psychiatric unit may become complete service.
In other districts, the mental hospital will continue to have supportive role.
Need to avoid two-tier system in which mental hospital remains under-privileged.

Need to define type of patient appropriate for mental hospital of the future: these might include EMI, new long stay and old long-stay, special units.
Joint planning between Health Authorities and Social Services crucial.

PROVISION OF SECURITY

Patient should only be placed in conditions of special security when strictly necessary and no alternatives possible.

Regional security units
Recommended by Butler Committee and DHSS.
   Care of patients who need greater supervision than the open-door system can provide, yet do not require security in one of the special hospitals.
   Butler Committee expressed concern at lack of appropriate local provision for this type of patient: pointed out that many offenders are sent to prison instead of hospital as a result. About one quarter of prisoners have significant mental disturbance.
   To be financed from central government funds, recent arrangements to provide revenue as well as capital support.
   Selection of patients under discussion.
   Variety of regimes: some provide locked door security, others use open door policy with high staff/patient ratio.
   Local forensic psychiatric service essential to provide early assessment and constant support in parallel with regional security unit.
   Special hospital provision of extra security for mentally-disturbed patients and offenders 20/ million general population or a total nationally of about 2000 beds.

FURTHER READING

DHSS (1975) *Better Services for the Mentally Ill*, London: HMSO.
DHSS/Home Office (1975) Report of the Committee on Mentally Abnormal Offenders, London: HMSO.
Early, D. F. & Nicholas M. (1977) Dissolution of the mental hospitals. *Brit. J. Psychiat.*, **130**, 117–122.
Mann & Cree W. (1975) The 'new long stay' in mental hospitals. *Brit. J. Hosp. Med.*, July, 56–63.

D. TERMINATION OF PREGNANCY

THE ABORTION ACT 1967

Termination permissible if
a) continuation of pregnancy would involve risk to the life of the pregnant woman, or of injury to her physical and mental health

or that of any existing children of her family, greater than if the
pregnancy was terminated.
b) there is a substantial risk that if the child was born, if would
suffer from such physical or mental abnormality as to be
seriously handicapped.
   The pregnant woman's actual or reasonably foreseeable
environment can be taken into account in reaching a decision.

ASSESSMENT PROBLEMS

Guilt and regret after termination is most common in those women
who show the most severe psychiatric disturbance at the time
abortion is requested.
   In a series of women refused abortion, 73% subsequently
satisfied with decision.
   In women who received abortions 25% self reproachful.
   Remember that termination of pregnancy is not without risks
(especially infection and haemorrhage) mortality 0.6 per 1000.
   Risks much increased after 12 weeks gestation.

PSYCHIATRIC INDICATIONS FOR TERMINATION

In the mother
1. History of recurrent puerperal psychosis or of one intractible
   puerperal illness especially if schizophrenic in type: high risk of
   recurrence with further pregnancy.
2. Acute emotional upset with suicide risk. 20% threaten suicide
   though it is rare in women refused abortion. Unwise to ignore,
   assess carefully, preferably in hospital, especially when severe
   depressive symptoms such as morbid guilt are present or
   recurrent self injury under stress.
3. Chronic mental illness, especially disabling schizophrenic
   psychosis.
4. Mental subnormality. Poor standard of care of existing children,
   especially when a further child might mean family breakdown.

In the child
Rubella in first 20 weeks of pregnancy.
Maternal smallpox, vaccination, exposure to cytotoxic drugs or
X-rays. (30 rads or more to pelvis within first trimester).
Familial illness (pheylketonuria, galactosaemia, haemophilia,
Christmas disease).
Chromosomal defects: mongolism (1 in 70 chance of a second
mongol child occurring in a family with one child already affected:
increased risk in older mothers).

FURTHER READING

Granville-Grossman, K. (1971) *Recent Advances in Clinical Psychiatry–1*
p. 266–280. Edinburgh: Churchill Livingstone.

E. INFANTILE AUTISM AND OTHER CHILD PSYCHOSES

SCHIZOPHRENIA

Occurs most often during adolescence: onset may be as early as 7 years of age.
Symptomatology identical with that in adults. 10% parents schizophrenic.
Excess of boys.
Childhood precursors of adult schizophrenia include: poor academic attainment, social isolation, personality oddities, I.Q. slightly below average.

DISINTEGRATIVE PSYCHOSIS

Normal up to 3rd and 4th year, when profound regression and behaviour disintegration occurs. Loss of speech, language, social skills, interest in objects, development of stereotypes and mannerisms.
    Occasionally follows measles, encephalitis or similar illness but usually no clear precipitating illness.

MANIC DEPRESSIVE PSYCHOSIS

Rare.

INFANTILE AUTISM

First described by Kanner in 1943. Generally regarded as being quite distinct from schizophrenia (occurs in infancy with low incidence of family schizophrenia, evidence of cerebral dysfunction, low I.Q., and has distinctive symptom pattern. Less likely to follow remitting pattern and rarely develop delusions and hallucinations in adulthood).

Prevalence
4 per 10 000 children have psychosis. Half of these comprise the specific syndrome of autism.

Symptoms and diagnostic criteria
Three kinds:
a) profound general failure to develop social and individual relationships.

b) language retardation (impaired comprehension, echolalia, pronominal reversal).

c) ritualistic compulsive phenomena (insistence on sameness) stereotyped, repetitive movement (especially hand and finger mannerisms).

short attention span, self injury, delayed bowel control.

Onset before 30 months. In 80% development has clearly been abnormal from birth.

I.Q. probably below average. 75% score in retarded range in spite of good motivation.

May be good rote memory and visuospatial function and these together with absence of physical stigmata, can be misleading in I.Q. assessment.

Fundamental defect may be a cognitive disorder involving language and central coding processes.

Pattern of scores on I.Q. tests different from those of mentally retarded children. Prognosis worse when I.Q. low.

Impaired social relationships
Lack of attachment behaviour and relative failure of bonding most marked in first five years (do not follow parents around the house, do not turn to them for comfort, nor distinguish between people).

Unusual use of eye to eye gaze.

Lack of cooperative group play, failure to make friendships, lack of empathy.

Says or does socially inappropriate things: gaucheness in later years prevents close relationships.

Language and other skills
Impaired imitation or meaningful use of objects and lack of imaginative play.

Babble speech abnormal (usually present in 2 year old).

Impaired comprehension of spoken language especially if it involves 2 or more ideas.

Lack gesture and mime.

Pronominal reversal ('you' instead of 'I') and echolalia. Unusual use of words and metaphors.

Talks less than normal.

In later years speech may lack cadence and inflexion and may seem pedantic and formal.

Insistence on sameness
Rigid, limited play patterns, lacking imagination.

Resist change in environment.

Intense attachment to toys and other objects.

Unusual preoccupation which excludes others (bus routes, train timetables, patterns, colours, numbers).

Ask stereotyped questions which require fixed answers.
Obsessional symptoms may develop later.

Variety of other behaviour
Feeding difficulties in infancy, stereotypies of hands, spinning of
whole body or objects, self injury.

Causes
Likely to be a behavioural syndrome without a single cause but
with common biological causation: may include several distinct
syndromes.
   Some type of cognitive deficit likely (use of language as above).
   Organic brain defect suggested in retarded autistics because 28%
of these later develop epilepsy in adolescence.
   Radiological studies suggest enlargement of temporal horn:
possible medial temporal lobe pathology.
   Increased incidence of non specific EEG abnormalities.
   Cytogenetic and biochemical: no consistent abnormality
demonstrated.
   Concordance in twins high in those without evidence of organic
brain dysfunction.
   Autism may be common in hypsarrhythmia, mental retardation
and sensory deficit secondary to congenital rubella.

Treatment
Few recover completely but treatment can in many lead to
improvement and social adjustment.
   Recent trend away from insight directed psychotherapy with
child towards:
   — facilitating normal social and linguistic development in spite
     of congenital defect.
   — avoidance of secondary handicaps.
   — emphasis on treating pre-school child.
   — helping total family.
   — special educational provision (systematic rather than
     permissive approach probably better. Poor response
     associated with low I.Q.).
   — drugs used symptomatically e.g. major tranquillisers for
     behaviour control.
   — behavioural techniques can be useful (operant or
     desensitation useful in reducing deviant disruptive
     behaviour).

PROGNOSIS

60% remain severely handicapped and totally unable to lead
independent life.

16% make good social adjustment and obtain a job (most remain eccentric with poor relationships).
24% intermediate outcome.
28% develop epilepsy (closely related to low I.Q.).

Indicators of poor outcome
Low I.Q. the most important, though a substantial proportion of intelligent autistic children do not do well.
Failure to acquire language by 5 years.
Severe behaviour disturbance in early childhood.
Disrupted disharmonious home.

FURTHER READING

Kolvin, I & Macmillan, A (1976) Child psychiatry. In *Recent Advances in Clinical Psychiatry–2*. ed. K. Granville-Grossman. Edinburgh: Churchill Livingstone.
Rutter, M. (1977) Infantile autism and other child psychoses. In *Child Psychiatry*. ed. Rutter & Hersov. Oxford: Blackwell Scientific.

F. ENURESIS

DEFINITION

Difficult to select point at which this becomes abnormal because prevalence curve shows smooth decline with increasing age.
Poussaint and Ditman: Nocturnal enuresis may be defined as nocturnal bedwetting in a child in whom the act of voiding otherwise occurs in the normal way.
This does not cover diurnal enuresis in which child is wet day and night.
Werry: Wetting in the school age period. This definition is useful because prevalence low at this age, spontaneous remission low, and child likely to be concerned at it.

TYPES

Primary (or continuous): never been dry.
Secondary (or onset): dry for at least a year then wet again.

EPIDEMIOLOGY

Prevalence at 5 years 17% (N.E. England), 10% (Stockholm), 32% Negroes in Baltimore.
Associated with social handicap in family.
Prevalence higher in boys than girls.

CAUSAL THEORIES

Physical or physiological

Sensitive period for emergence of dryness. Most children establish this between 18–54 months. Any interference with bladder control during this sensitive period might mean that child will be without control for a number of years.

.*Genetic.* MZ twins twice as concordant as DZ. Well known high familial incidence may be related to family custom.

Functional bladder capacity (as opposed to structural capacity). Failure of ability to hold urine for increasing periods in the day with extension into sleeping state.

Deep sleep pattern. Little evidence for this, either EEG or otherwise.

Developmental delay. Consistent with tendency to spontaneous remission with increasing age, higher incidence in low birth weight children, poorer physical growth in enuretics, excess of boys (in common with other developmental disorders).

Physical factors. Urinary infection (in 10% of girls who wet nightly). Little consistent association with urinary tract defects.

Learning theory explanations.
Nocturnal continence probably achieved by complementary action of neurophysiological maturity and learning processes.

Poor social conditions and training. Low I.Q. may impair learning.

Psychodynamic
Increased incidence of psychological disturbance in enuretics especially in girls, but 70% are without psychiatric difficulties.

No association of enuresis with any specific syndrome.

Anxiety provoked by stress may lead to bladder irritability and hence impede learnt bladder control in predisposed children.

No specificity of stress demonstrated.

Need to distinguish early adverse factors from later perpetuating ones: Douglas found excess of stress at age 3 years in enuretics.

VARIETIES OF ENURESIS

Newcastle. Primary type: primarily biological basis. Secondary type: psychogenic.

Maudsley. Nocturnal (more common in boys), mainly developmental and biological. Diurnal (more common in girls) associated with behaviour disorder.

TREATMENT

Guidance for parents, helping stressed families.
Minimise over-critical or punishing parental attitudes.

Encourage success.

Lifting 2 – 3 hours after going to bed.

Fluid restriction in evenings.

Bell and pad technique may help some: effects more persistent than antidepressants.

Psychotherapy effective only when there is good evidence of associated emotional disorder.

Antidepressant medication e.g. Imipramine. May act by anticholinegic effect, though long term follow up suggests that relapse likely as soon as it is stopped. Potentially toxic and if no response in 4 weeks, discontinue.

Chlordiazepoxide when anxiety high.

Better response to drugs:

— secondary enuresis

— other milestones achieved normally

— no family history of enuresis.

FURTHER READING

Kolvin, I. & Macmillan, A. (1976) Child psychiatry. In *Recent Advances in Clinical Psychiatry – 2*. ed. Granville-Grossman, K. Edinburgh: Churchill Livingstone.

G. THE PSYCHIATRY OF ADOLESCENCE

Exact age range ill-defined: 12 – 19 year olds comprise 11.5% of population (5.3 million). The major experience during adolescence is one of transition.

Puberty marks the onset of adolescence. In girls there is a critical weight at which the pubertal sequence is triggered off: to be precise this is when body fat increases to 22% of total body weight (Frisch & Revelle 1971). During the last 150 years the menarche has occurred progressively earlier by 4 months per decade in Western Europe. In childhood there is a powerful negative feedback of gonadal hormones on the hypothalamus. In puberty there is a reduction in feedback with resulting increased secretion of gonadotrophins by the anterior pituitary. In girls in late puberty a positive feedback mechanism appears whereby oestrogen stimulates gonadotrophin release in mid menstrual cycle, leading to ovulation.

Physical changes

In boys growth spurt begins at 13 years (maximum at 14).

In girls growth spurt begins at 10 – 11 years (maximum at 11 – 12).

Considerable individual variation. Sexual maturation closely linked, tends to occur 18 – 24 months later in boys. Menarche occurs after the peak velocity of growth spurt.

Psychological changes
Maturation of logical reasoning and ability to look at problems from a variety of perspectives utilising abstract concepts. Major changes in the way the world is conceptualised. Piaget: Change from concrete operational to abstract logic and reasoning.

Strives towards independence, frequently associated with ambivalence and rejection of adult values.

Intense examination of capabilities and goals (identity crisis — Erikson).

Adolescence has only recently become a prolonged intermediate period of education and peer group activities between childhood and adult life.

Social changes
Altered expectation from others (academic, job).

Expectation of conformity with peer group and conflict with parents.

COMMON SYMPTOMS

Rutter (Isle of Wight study of 14 years old) showed that minor conflicts with parents were common. Severe family conflict always needs assessment in case intervention may help.

21% of 14 year olds were found to have psychiatric disorder but in only 10% was this obvious to adults.

Alienation from parents more frequent in those with psychiatric disorder. Leslie (industrial town, N. England) 12–16 year olds: 6% boys, 3% girls severe handicapping psychiatric disorder, 15% boys, 11% girls moderate disorder.

Anxiety and depressive feelings occur in about half of normal adolescents. May be marked lability of mood.

May over-react to stress and appear egocentric in attitude. Incur conflict with parents who see them as selfish and inconsiderate.

SYNDROMES IN ADOLESCENCE

Conduct disorder
A persistent picture of antisocial symptoms usually combined with abnormal interpersonal relationships.

More common in boys, especially from unstable, unhappy families. Often associated with reading difficulties.

Promiscuity and extra marital pregnancy in girls.

Testing-out common: push others to the limit of tolerance or further.

Neurosis
Anxiety, phobias, depression.
 Preoccupation with relationship difficulties and sexual/bodily functions.
  School refusal.
  Anorexia nervosa.

Suicide
Rare in adolescence but more common than in children.
? more common in adolescents of high I.Q. and above average stature.

Attempted suicide
7–10% of referrals to child psychiatric clinics are for the threatened or attempted suicide (Shaffer).

Psychosis
Insidious onset of schizophrenia during adolescence may denote poor prognosis.

Drugs and alcohol abuse
Experimentation may begin in adolescence.

TREATMENT

Referral rates tend to be low even though psychiatric disorders slightly more common than in adults.
 ? related to reluctance to seek help.
 Specialist approach geared to adolescents' needs is justified: facilities for younger ones need to be different from those for older ones.
 4 beds per 100 000 required for younger adolescents.
 Need to work with entire family (e.g. setting goals).
 Adolescent units need close links with schools and the community especially voluntary agencies.
 Variety of approaches being explored.
 Family therapy particularly useful in adolescence:
   — brings all relevant information into the open.
   — other family members need help when adolescent member has problems.
   — prevents obstructive resistance from relatives.
   — dilutes adolescent's hostility to therapist.
   — helps family to tolerate adolescent.
   — may prevent unnecessary hospital admission.

FURTHER READING

Brugger, P. & Davies, G. (1977) Family therapy in adolescent psychiatry. *Brit. J. Psychiat.*, **131**, 433–447.

DHSS (1975) *Better Services for the Mentally Ill: Adolescents.* pp. 58–61. London: HMSO.

Wolkind, S. N. & Coleman, J. C. (1976) The psychiatry of adolescence. *Brit. J. Hosp. Med.*, June **15**, 575–582.

H. NON-ACCIDENTAL INJURY IN CHILDREN

Kempe in 1962 coined the term 'battered baby'.

CAUSES

A description of behaviour which may be due to a variety of causes.
May be related to:
— a wish to eliminate an encumbrance.
— a wish to relieve suffering.
— disordered thinking in mentally ill parent.
— displacement of anger, frustration, or retaliation.
— a problem in the child itself.

INCIDENCE

Major injury: 1 in 1000 children under 4 years per annum England and Wales.

About 2–4% of children in subnormality hospitals are brain damaged because of assault, usually by violent shaking or battering.

About 25% of severely attacked children are intellectually damaged as a result.

CLINICAL FEATURES

Found in all social classes.

Parents may vary greatly in intelligence, attractiveness, mental stability, personality and apparent efficiency in running the home.

In the child

Evidence of successive injuries especially bruises of different ages. Bizarre injuries.

All fractures in children up to 2 years of age should be viewed with suspicion.

Non-accidental poisoning with drugs: may cause behavioural changes which are sometimes bizarre: parents may abuse drugs themselves.

May be fearful towards adults or show over-anxious concern for the parents' welfare. Often unhappy.

In the parents
May be evasive, provide contradictory information, lack warmth
towards child, lack confidence in handling it, or express overt
criticism e.g. its refusal to be comforted, or its excessive crying.

FACTORS PREVENTING EARLY DIAGNOSIS

Incomplete and misinterpreted facts
Ignorance of what to look for and ask, shortage of time, fear of
arousing anger or litigation, wish to maintain confidentially, being
deceived by parents who may be plausible and misleading.

Available but uncollected information
Mobility of family, deliberate change of doctor or hospital to
conceal successive assaults, inaccurate identification of the child
concerned, lack of standardised records, failure to make one person
responsible for collation of information (key worker).

Unavailable information
Concealment in privacy of home (neighbour may be useful
informant): the tradition of protecting the client may obscure the
needs of the child.

PREVENTION AND TREATMENT

Good and immediate communication between different branches
of caring services essential.
    Regional and Area Review Committees set up for this purpose.
    Case registers a further important development.
    When a suspect case arises, a conference of all helping persons
is called and further action agreed by group decision. Key worker
nominated as integrator.
    If child at immediate risk, may need urgent admission to hospital
for assessment and treatment. Occasionally when child in danger
and parents object, it may be necessary to remove it compulsorily
under a Place of Safety order.

FURTHER READING

Rogers, D. et al. (1976) Non-accidental poisoning: an extended syndrome
    of child abuse. *Brit. Med. J.*, **1**, 793–796.
Working Party of the Royal College of Psychiatrists (1977) *Brit. J. Psychiat.*,
    131, 366–380.

1. MANAGEMENT OF THE VIOLENT PATIENT

Each hospital should have a clear written policy.

All staff must accept responsibility to intervene in any situation where a person may suffer injury: adequate training of medical and nursing staff essential.

Prevention in ward community needs full cooperation between medical and nursing personnel.

The consultant or his deputy should be available at the earliest opportunity following a violent incident for full evaluation and appropriate management.

Potentially violent individuals should only be admitted to wards that have sufficient staff (1:1 recommended by RC Psychiatrists and COHSE).

Avoid excess concentration of difficult patients in one ward especially when it has inadequate facilities.

Emphasis should be on prevention: maintain good ward atmosphere, adequate staff communications and morale. COHSE critical of medical staff attitudes.

Avoid unduly restrictive regime, ensure adequate occupational therapy, preferably away from the ward for part of each day for special group activity.

Note premonitory signs (know patients well).

The violent episode
Establish diagnosis (e.g. alcohol withdrawal states, epileptic episodes).
Staff remain calm and non-critical.
Avoid physical confrontation if possible. Talk and listen to patient.
Need sufficient staff to control outburst without leading to injury.
If restraint necessary use minimal degree of force to control violence, aim to calm rather than provoke.
Use clothing rather than direct bodily restraint if possible but may have to hold hair if patient biting. Never press on neck, chest or abdomen.
Remove patient's shoes.
Great care if intramuscular injection given.
Separate for minimal period, with medical agreement.

Report on violent incidents
Ensure that adequate report is made (as a minimal procedure — in ward report, nursing and medical notes).
Time, place.
Factual account.
Action taken.
Names of all involved.

Description of patient's medical state.
Direction of aggression.
Injury and damage done.

Nursing Officer responsible for further reporting in the hospital. If actual injury serious or damage to property, copy sent to District Health Authority.

Injured staff may qualify for Industrial Injury Benefit or Criminal Injuries Compensation, (advice sought from DHA immediately).

FURTHER READING

The Management of Violent and Potentially Violent Patients in Hospital. DHSS HC(76)11. London:HMSO

PART II

Neurology and neurophysiology in relation to psychiatry

Common clinical problems

A. HEADACHE

Structures sensitive to pain include all extracranial tissues, and intracranial tissues such as basal dura and pia mater, venous sinuses, arteries of the circle of Willis, and nerves with sensory afferents. Brain tissue is insensitive to pain.

TYPES

1. Tension
Description: related to scalp muscle contraction; usually generalised; duration hours; throbbing, clamping, stabbing; scalp tender.
 Treatment: reassurance, analgesics, alleviation of anxiety.

2. Migraine
Description: episodic disorder of function of cranial blood vessels, with unilateral or generalised headache. Often accompanied by nausea, may be preceded or accompanied by transient focal neurological symptoms (e.g. hemiplegic, opthalmoplegic and basilar migraine), female preponderance, often familial.
 Investigations: if diagnosis is in doubt, skull X-ray, CAT scan.
 Treatment of the attack: analgesics. Ergotamine (if no severe vascular disease).
 Prophylaxis: intermittent courses of tranquillisers, particularly if situational stress. May need to stop contraceptive pill. Clonidine (dixarit) 25 to 150 μg daily. Pizotifen (Sanomigran) 0.5 mg, usually three a day. Migraleve (buclizine, codeine, paracetamol mixture), 2 tabs at night. Methysergide 2–6 mg daily, restricted course only.

3. Migrainous neuralgia (cluster headache)
Description: episodic, severe pain in eye and face, often at night. Associated with conjunctival suffusion, lacrimation. Duration ½–2 hours: repeated over several weeks, interspersed with prolonged periods of freedom.
 Treatment: oral ergotamine 1–2 mg nightly as preventive.

4. Raised intracranial pressure
Description: paroxysmal, throbbing, bilateral occipital or frontal; aggravated by coughing, bending, straining; worse on waking. May be associated with vomiting. Usually but not necessarily papilloedema. May be transient obscurations of vision and/or diplopia due to VI nerve lesion.

Investigations: skull X-ray — erosion of dorsum sellae; copper beaten appearance of vault and suture diastasis in children. Chest X-ray. Routine blood count. CAT scan. May also need further investigation in special unit, e.g. angiography, contrast encephalography.

5. Low intracranial pressure (relatively rare)
Can arise after lumbar puncture, skull fracture, subdural haematoma, or spontaneously. Severe on standing, relieved by lying. There may be meningism, vomiting.

Treatment: of the cause, and if necessary, saline infusion.

6. Infective (e.g. meningitis, encephalitis, abscess, thrombophlebitis)
Description: generalised, constant, may be meningism, focal CNS signs. Fever.

Investigations: blood count, ESR or viscosity. Chest, skull X-rays. Lumbar puncture *providing there is no* papilloedema, and *no* suspicion of local intracranial lesion.

Treatment: appropriate to the organism and/or local cause.

7. Post traumatic
Description: generalised, variable duration, worse on bending and with alcohol.

Investigations: skull X-ray, EEG, CAT scan if subdural haematoma suspected (progressive intellectual or memory deficit, variable confusion or disorientation, or focal signs).

8. Toxic
e.g. alcohol, carbon monoxide poisoning, oral contraceptives. Usually clear evidence with careful history.

9. Haemorrhage
a. Subarachnoid
Description: sudden very severe headache in an otherwise fit person. Can be precipitated by straining, exertion. Diffuse or occipital. Usually vomiting, may be clouding of consciousness, meningism, and/or focal CNS signs. 10% have fundal haemorrhages.

Investigations: lumbar puncture, unless papilloedema or focal signs. CAT scan. Angiography to locate site of bleed — needs specialist assessment.

b. *Intracerebral*
Sudden, severe, with altered consciousness; focal signs common.

10. Hypertensive
Not a common association, but may occur. In acute crises can occur with vomiting. Duration few minutes to hours. Associated optic fundal and cardiac changes.

11. Cervical spondylosis
Occipital, radiating forwards. Duration hours to days. Precipitated by certain positions of head. Can be caused by whiplash injury.
    Investigations: X-ray cervical spine.

12. Opthalmologic causes
Anomalies of refraction. Acute glaucoma: often frontal; vomiting, bradycardia, visual impairment.

13. Cranial arteritis
Constant, localised over temporal, facial and/or occipital arteries. Localised tenderness. Maybe focal CNS signs because of involvement of intracranial vessels. Danger — loss of vision.
    Investigations: blood count, ESR or plasma viscosity. Local biopsy of vessel.
    Treatment: urgent. Prednisolone unless specific contraindications.

FURTHER READING

Bickerstaff, E. R. (1975) Migraine and facial pain. *Medicine,* **34**, 2054–2064.

B. FACIAL PAIN

1. LOCAL PATHOLOGY

Affecting teeth, sinuses, ear, nose, throat, as well as orbital cavity and superior orbital fissure.
    Description: pain of variable nature and site.
    Investigations: clinical examination; X-rays of skull, orbit, sinuses.

2. FACIAL NEURALGIAS

a. Trigeminal neuralgia
Description: age of onset usually more than 60 years (exceptions V nerve tumours and multiple sclerosis — both rare). Unilateral, stereotyped, severe paroxysms of lancinating pain over localised area of face. Recurrent bursts, with periods of freedom. Relapses and remissions. 'Trigger zones', pain precipitated by stimulation of

sensitive areas of the face or gums or by speaking, swallowing, chewing.

Usually affects 2nd and 3rd division first, and later 1st division. No abnormal signs unless symptomatic of local nerve lesion.

Treatment: carbamazepine (Tegretol) up to 6 × 200 mg daily, or phenytoin (Epanutin) up to 300 mg daily, or clonazepam (Rivotril) up to 3 × 200 mg daily (carbamazepine usually most effective). Local injection of nerve branches may be needed for unresponsive cases, and very rarely an injection or operation on the ganglion itself.

b. Auriculotemporal neuralgia (rare)
Usually after lesion in parotid gland. Chewing provokes burning pain, local redness of skin, profuse local sweating in preauricular region.

c. Nasociliary neuralgia (rare)
Episodic or prolonged pain in nasal region, inner canthus and eyeball, with local suffusion. Local trigger zones. Exclude local inflammatory causes and occasional associated aneurysm of carotid.

d. Glossopharyngeal neuralgia (rare)
Paroxysms of severe pain, or prolonged. Unilateral affection of tongue, tonsillar area and pharynx. May radiate to the ear. Precipitated by swallowing, moving tongue, talking. Trigger zones in pharynx.

e. Geniculate neuralgia
Lancinating pains in preauricular region, ear, palate, maxilla, mastoid area, may be abnormality of taste and excessive salivation. Can occur with herpes of geniculate ganglion and facial palsy (Ramsay-Hunt syndrome) — cutaneous vesicles in the ear and over mastoid area.

f. Neuralgia of other nerves (rare)
Superior laryngeal nerve, with unilateral hypothyroid pain; auricular branch of vagus nerve with suboccipital pain; Sluder's neuralgia — local nasal pain due to lesion of pterygopalatine ganglion.

g. Raeder's paratrigeminal neuralgia
Severe pain in and around one eye, plus Horner's syndrome. Continuous progressively severe pain, often due to local malignancy at base of skull.

h. Costen's syndrome

Shooting pain in mandible and temple, triggered only by chewing or talking.

Treatment: adjustment of bite by orthodontic procedures.

3. MIGRAINOUS NEURALGIA (see Headache)

4. ATYPICAL FACIAL NEURALGIA

Description: unilateral, diffuse, burning facial pain. Prolonged duration, occasionally associated with facial flushing. Usually affects middle-aged females, who may also be depressed. *N.B.* Exclude local causes e.g. carious teeth, infected sinuses.

Treatment: extremely difficult, usually defies analgesics, ergotamine and antidepressants.

5. POST HERPETIC NEURALGIA

Pain after local herpes zoster infection. Commonly affects 1st division V nerve. Continuous burning pain. Affects elderly, who may also become depressed.

Treatment: local friction. Analgesics. Avoid addictive drugs.

6. CRANIAL ARTERITIS

Granulomatous arteritis affecting elderly. Pain in face, jaw, and/or mouth. Worse on eating. Headache — see above. Tender over superficial arteries.

May be also muscle pain, tenderness and proximal limb girdle weakness. *N.B.* Visual loss may be sudden and irreversible.

Diagnostic: temporal artery biopsy. Raised ESR. Serum $\propto_2$ globulin increased, albumin reduced.

Treatment: initial high doses steroids. Maintenance dose 6 months-1 year, dependent on ESR.

7. MYOCARDIAL ISCHAEMIA

Pain in lower jaw, neck, often related to exertion.

FURTHER READING

Bickerstaff, E. R. (1975) Migraine and facial pain. *Medicine,* **34**, 2054.

C. INVOLUNTARY MOVEMENTS

1. TREMOR

Rhythmic sinusoidal movement, maximal when:
a) Limb at rest — 'rest tremor'
Examples: Parkinson's disease, parkinsonism, rarely cerebral tumours, drugs e.g. reserpine, tetrabenazine, phenothiazines, butyrophenones.
b) Limb outstretched against gravity — 'postural tremor'.
Examples: physiological, exaggerated physiological in anxiety states, thyrotoxicosis, alcoholism, drugs e.g. trycyclics, bronchodilators, heavy metal poisoning, benign essential (often familial) tremor, cerebellar lesions, Wilson's disease, neurosyphilis.
c) During voluntary movement — 'intention tremor'.
Examples: cerebellar or brain stem lesions due to multiple sclerosis, spinocerebellar degenerations, tumours or vascular disease.

2. a. CHOREA

Brief, random, irregular, jerky movements of face, tongue, limbs and trunk. May be followed by voluntary movement in same direction to mask the affliction. Walking can be affected (lurching, stopping, dancing-type gait). Limbs may be hypotonic, power is normal, reflexes retained, flexor plantar responses.
Examples: a) Sydenham's chorea — children or young adults, can recur in later pregnancy. May be unilateral — hemichorea.
b) Huntington's chorea — (with dementia). Autosomal dominant inheritance or sporadic. Onset 30–40 years, progressive. Onset in childhood as an akinetic-rigid Parkinsonian syndrome.
c) Chorea can also occur in thyrotoxicosis, systemic lupus erythematosis, polycythemia rubra vera, encephalitis lethargica, or be induced by drugs e.g. phenytoin.

b. BALLISMUS OR HEMIBALLISMUS

Sudden, wild limb movements, caused by vascular lesion in contralateral subthalamic nucleus, usually slow spontaneous recovery.

3. MYOCLONUS

Brief, shock-like contractions of muscle groups, causing sudden limb movements. Irregular or rhythmic, often repetitive in some muscles.

Seen in:

Idiopathic epilepsy

Progressive myoclonic epilepsy:
— familial
— Lafora body disease
— lipidoses
— spino cerebellar degenerations.

Metabolic disorders:
— renal failure
— hepatic failure
— respiratory failure
— alcohol and drug withdrawal.

Structural brain disease:
— post-anoxic
— Creutzfeldt-Jakob disease
— subacute sclerosing leuco-encephalitis
— encephalitis lethargica.

4. TICS

Brief repetitive muscle contractions, invariably stereotyped. Can be controlled with effort. Very common in young children, may persist to adulthood in a few subjects. Specific treatment rarely required. May be severe, associated with repetitive swearing in Gilles de la Tourette's syndrome in childhood.

5. TORSION DYSTONIA (athetosis)

Sustained, irregular, semirotatory muscle spasms distorting the body into characteristic postures e.g. torticollis, retrocollis, lordosis, scoliosis, arm extension, foot plantar flexion and inversion.

Initially with action, later at rest, maybe resulting persistent limb deformity.

a) Symptomatic in:
— cerebral palsy
— Wilson's disease
— Juvenile Huntington's chorea
— Hallevorden-Spatz disease
— encephalitis lethargica.

b) Drugs: phenothiazines, butyrophenones, metclopramide, diazoxide.

c) Idiopathic dystonia musculorum deformans (onset in children or adults, intellect normal, cause uncertain).

d) Paroxysmal dystonia — paroxysmal choreoathetosis.

6. LOCALISED INVOLUNTARY MOVEMENTS

a) Hemifacial spasm: brief, unilateral, irregular contractions of facial muscles. Most — no cause, but can follow Bell's Palsy, or indicate VII nerve compression.
b) Blepharospasm: affects orbicularis oculi. Usually idiopathic, most commonly in elderly patients. Also symptomatic in Parkinson's disease or torsion dystonia.
c) Spasmodic torticollis: *Idiopathic* — most common. Age 30–50 years, painful neck, resistant to treatment.
   Symptomatic — (trauma or infection of cervical spine, cerebellar tumour in children, drugs e.g. phenothiazines).
d) Writer's cramp: specific inability to write, type or play musical instrument. Resistant to most treatments. Minor tranquillisers and retraining may help in a few.
e) Dyskinesias: tardive e.g. facial, often with chorea of digitis and dystonic trunk movements. Complicate phenothiazine and butyrophenone medication.

7. AKITHISIA

Inability to keep lower limbs still: restless shuffling movements. May accompany drug induced parkinsonism in phenothiazine and butyrophenone medication.

FURTHER READING

Marsden, D. (1975) *Medicine*. **35**, 2146–2156.

D. THE PARKINSONIAN SYNDROME

Characterised by degenerative pathological changes affecting the pigmented nuclei of the brain stem. Nerve cells in the substantia nigra, globus pallidus, and corpus striatum show atrophy and loss of pigmentation. In the idiopathic form there may be prominent eosinophilic intracytoplasmic inclusions — Lewy bodies.

CAUSES

A. Idiopathic
Parkinson's disease (Paralysis Agitans)
   60 000–80 000 patients in U.K.
   Prevalence: 1 in 1000, rising over age of 50 to 1 in 200.

B. Parkinson's syndrome — Parkinsonism
 1. Post encephalitic, e.g. after epidemic encephalitis lethargica in 1920s but sporadic since.
 2. Arteriosclerotic: often unilateral, rigid-akinetic syndrome,

tremor less frequent. Age usually above 60 years, other signs of arteriosclerosis, e.g. mental, pseudo bulbar palsy or other neurological signs.
3. In certain heredo-familial degenerative disorders, e.g. olivoponto-cerebellar atrophy, Wilson's disease, Huntington's chorea (rigid form), Guam Island dementia and parkinsonian complex.
4. Associated with more diffuse organic brain disease:
   a) senile dementia, presenile dementia, e.g. Alzheimer's disease, Creutzfeld-Jacob disease.
   b) post anoxic, poisoning and drugs, e.g. carbon monoxide, carbon disulphide, sulphur dioxide, butyrophenones, reserpine.
   c) tumour — rare.
   d) polycythaemia.
   e) progressive supranuclear palsy, with paralysis of ocular movements. Sporadic or familial, age 50–70 years. Usually also dementia, rarely pyramidal and cerebellar signs.
   f) post traumatic — very rare. Occasionally after single severe episode with permanent brain damage, or after recurrent less severe injuries, e.g. boxers.

SYMPTOMS AND SIGNS

1. Akinesia
Inhibition of primary automatic movements. Loss of facial expression, lack of blinking and other associated expressive movements, loss of normal arm swinging when walking. Festinating gait — small shuffling steps, pro and retropulsion.

2. Rigidity
Increased tone of extrapyramidal type:
a) 'lead-pipe', present throughout passive movements of a limb.
b) resting tone increased, and increase in antagonistic muscle tone.
c) cog-wheel phenomenon — stepwise variation in tone with passive alternating movements of pronation/supination or flexion/extension.
d) postural abnormality — bent forwards, knees and elbows flexed. May lead to skeletal deformities.

3. Tremor
Rhythmic, sinusoidal movements of a limb at frequency 4–8 per second. Typically maximal at rest, abolished by voluntary movement, but can persist as action tremor. Increased by emotion, abolished in sleep. Finger tremor — 'pill rolling'.

4. Other physical changes
(*N.B.* normal reflexes, flexor plantar responses if uncomplicated).
Micrographia.
Quiet monotonous voice; poor articulation, word repetition
(echolalia).
Respiratory abnormality (irregular frequency and depth).
Accentuated nasopalpebral reflex — positive glabellar tap sign.
Autonomic symptoms (especially post-encephalitic, seborrhoea,
dribbling, sweating attacks).
Oculogyric crises (post encephalitic and drug induced). Fixed
upward deviation of eyes for minutes or hours, occasionally also
head tilting.

5. Mental changes
Initially usually none. Later apathy, emotional lability (especially
with supranuclear palsy), depression. Dementia when complicating
brain disease. *N.B.* Acute confusional states, hallucinations, apathy,
lethargy, can be drug induced or herald intercurrent infection.

TREATMENT

Medical

a. Drugs

1. *Laevodopa.* Originally given alone, now usually in combination
with a selective extracerebral decorboxylase inhibitor. Latter
prevents conversion of dopa to dopamine outside the brain, but
fails to enter brain tissues, so allows increased efficacy of lower
dose within the brain. Reduces side effects. Sinemet 275 (250 mg L.
Dopa, 25 mg carbidopa). Sinemet 110 (L. Dopa 100 mg, carbidopa
10 mg), dose: up to 6×275. Madopar (100 mg L. Dopa, 25 mg
benserazide), dose: up to 6 a day.
    Side effects: nausea, vomiting, weight loss, hypotension.
                involuntary movements — dose related.
                psychiatric complications such as confusional state
                (in 25%), but remits with reduced dose.
                contraindicated with monoamine oxidase
                inhibitors, in recent myocardial infarction, and may
                exacerbate glaucoma.

2. *Amantadine*: (Symmetrel) 100 mg bd or tds. Initially moderately
potent but effect may diminish. Reduce dose slowly to avoid
rebound effects. Side effects — ankle oedema, skin changes,
confusional states.

3. *Anticholinergics,* e.g. benzhexol (Artane, Pipanol) up to 15 mg
daily.

orphenadrine (Disipal) up to 400 mg daily.

benztropine (Cogentin) up to 6 mg daily —
moderate effect on rigidity, akinesia, less
effect on tremor.

Side effects: dry mouth, blurred vision, constipation, urinary
retention, confusional state.

4. *Bromocriptine* (directly acting dopamine agonist). More
prolonged action than L. Dopa.

5. *Propranolol.* Can help tremor.

6. *Physiotherapy.* Help with walking and activities of daily living.
Often particularly useful in conjunction with phase of drug induced
improvement.

Surgical
Stereotactic operation.

Mechanical, chemical, electrical or cryogenic lesion in globus
pallidus to diminish rigidity, or in posterolateral nucleus of
thalamus to reduce tremor. A rare procedure since advent of L.
Dopa. Rigidity most likely to be helped, tremor less likely, and
akinesia least amenable.

Indications: unilateral disease, significant social disability,
unresponsive to full medication.

Contraindications: previous cerebrovascular accident,
hypertension, marked mental changes, relative contraindications,
age more than 65 years.

FURTHER READING

Mumenthaler, M. (1976). *Neurology.* Chicago: Thieme.

E. DEMENTIA — DIAGNOSIS AND INVESTIGATION

Dementia is a syndrome arising from cerebral disease; often
progressive; characterised by a decline of intellect and personality
which reflect a disturbance of memory, orientation, capacity for
conceptual thought and often of affect. Failure or impairment of
any mental function can occur in dementia, and selective deficits
imply focal dysfunction.

HISTORY

Essential to have objective information from relatives, friends and work colleagues to ascertain *change* from premorbid function, duration, speed of onset and evidence of selective difficulty. Family history, in case of inherited disorders, e.g. Huntington's chorea.

EXAMINATION

a) Full general physical for evidence of systemic disease, e.g. metabolic or neoplastic.
b) Neurological for focal cranial nerve or limb signs. *N.B.* Look for apraxia — a defect of action inexplicable by simple motor or sensory loss — implies parietal lobe involvment.
c) Simple tests of mental function
   1. Language:
      (i) naming objects:
         — *nomimal dysphasia* if single nouns.
         — *expressive dysphasia* if more extensive disability.
      (ii) spoken commands:
         — *receptive dysphasia* — failure to understand single words or sentences.
         — *dyslexia* — reading disability. If comprehension and speech intact, indicates dominant hemisphere parieto-occipital lesion.
         — *dysgraphia* — writing disorder.
   2. Calculation — 7s substracted serially from 100 (is also a test of concerntration).
         — *dyscalculia* — rare as a primary disorder.
   3. Spatial organisation — drawing a star or a cube.
   4. Short term memory — digit span, usually more than 5 forward.
   5. Problem solving — e.g. placing digits in reverse order.
   6. Recent memory — recalling current events. Babcock sentence or 3 unrelated words.
d) Where doubt remains and/or suspicion of selective deficits, then detailed psychometric assessment may be required.

INVESTIGATIONS

Hb, WBC, ESR (or plasma viscosity), W.R.
   Metabolic — urea, electrolytes, calcium, liver function tests, thyroid function, vitamin B_{12}.
   EEG — evidence of focal abnormality, serial records, monitor possible progression. May be normal, is *not* correlated with degree of intellectual disturbance.

CAT scan — evidence of atrophy, local or generalised.

If necessary, to investigate suspected neurological conditions, then arteriography, isotope encephalography, or very rarely air/contrast encephalography after specialist referral.

FURTHER READING

Miller, E. (1975) Psychometric assessment. *Brit. J. Hosp. Med. Supplement*, 267–272.

Pearce, J. & Miller, D. E. (1973) *Clinical Aspects of Dementia*. London: Balliere Tindall.

Warrington, E. K. & Gautier-Smith, P. C. (1975) Clinical assessment of higher cerebral function. *Medicine*, **35**, 2049–2053.

Neurological investigations

1. X-RAYS OF THE SKULL may show:

a) Fractures.
b) Localised or generalised alteration in skull thickness or local defects.
c) Abnormal shape, e.g. microcephaly, craniostenosis.
d) Signs of raised intracranial pressure: in childhood, suture diastasis, copper-beaten appearance (less reliable): in adults, may be erosion of dorsum sellae.
e) Abnormal vascular channels, e.g. in vascular anomalies and some neoplasms.
f) Displacement of a calcified pineal gland.
g) Calcification of intracranial blood vessels, or calcification in some neoplasms.
h) Abnormalities of skull base and cervical spine alignment (may require special views) as in Arnold Chiari malformation.
i) Localised views or tomograms may show specific areas of abnormality, e.g. widening of internal auditory meatus with acoustic neuroma.

2. X-RAYS OF THE VERTEBRAL COLUMN may show:

a) Fractures.
b) Abnormal curvature.
c) Abnormal local or generalised bony structure, e.g. neoplasm, osteoporosis.
d) Abnormal shape of vertebrae, e.g. collapse, osteophyte formation.
e) Abnormal intervertebral spaces or foramina, encroachment by osteophytes, or tumours such as neurofibromas.
f) Abnormal intervertebral joints.
g) Calcification of extracranial vessels.
h) Abnormalities of spinal canal, e.g. widening due to neoplasm, narrowing due to prolapsed intervertebral disc.

3. LUMBAR PUNCTURE

Indications

Investigation of suspected:
a) Meningitis:
   (i) infective
   (ii) carcinomatous.
b) Subarachnoid haemorrhage.
c) Neurosyphilis (repeated 6 months and 2 years following treatment)

As part of myelographic investigation to look at:
a) Spinal cord and roots.
b) Disc spaces.
c) Cerebrospinal pathways for evidence of local block.

In treatment: injection of drugs for:
a) Tuberculous or other bacterial meningitis.
b) Leukaemic infiltration of the meninges.

Contraindications
a) Raised intracranial pressure.
b) Suspected space occupying lesion in the posterior fossa.
c) Suspected intracranial space occupying lesion above the tentorium.
d) Presence of ventricular dilation and possible raised intracranial pressure.
e) Tissue suppuration near the puncture site.

4. CEREBROSPINAL FLUID CHANGES

	Normal range	Common abnormalities
Cells	less than 5 mm^3 (all lymphocytes)	Traumatic tap – blood clears in successive samples. Haemorrhage – uniformly blood-stained xanthochromia within 6 hours of a bleed, persists for three weeks. Cloudy fluid – if cells > 400/mm^3. Moderate increase in cells – trauma, recent air encephalogram, intracranial neoplasms. Marked increase in cells – bacterial (polymorphs) or viral (lymphocytes) meningitis, fungal infections.
Protein	15–45 mg% (infants up to 3 months normal limit up to 100 mg%)	a) *Increased up to several hundred mg% in* obstruction to C.S.F. pathways, may clot in tube (Froins' syndrome). b) *Albumino – cytologic dissociation (cells not increased markedly) may occur in:*

C.S.F. obstruction and in Guillain-Barré syndrome.

c) *Raised in:* Liver disorders, paraprotein-aemias, chronic encephalitides, neurosyphilis, multiple sclerosis. Immunoglobulin G fraction raised in some patients with multiple sclerosis. and neurosyphilis.

Glucose   50–80 mg%   *Raised in:* diabetes mellitus.
Reduced in: meningitis-carcinomatous (marked reduction). infective, (marked reduction). tuberculous (moderate reduction). abscess (moderate or severe reduction- cell count dependent).

5. RETINAL EXAMINATION WITH FLOURESCEIN ANGIOGRAPHY

To ascertain presence of papilloedema when doubt exists. Flourescein leaks from capillaries into extravascular tissues in the presence of disc oedema, and stains the peripapillary retina for up to 10 minutes; none leaks when disc is normal.

6. COMPUTERISED AXIAL TOMOGRAPHY (CAT SCAN)

Indicates:
a) Ventricular size and shape, e.g. hydrocephalus, cortical atrophy.
b) Pathological intracranial lesions (as small as 1 cm in diameter).
Reasonable assessment of:
a) Type of lesion, using tissue density measurements, e.g. infarction, haemorrhage, cystic lesions.
Intravenous contrast injections can increase the definition of some lesions, e.g. neoplasm.
May miss:
a) Diffuse early lesions, e.g. microgliomatosis.
b) Very small localised lesions.
c) Small lesions in certain critical areas, e.g. near the base of the skull, near the anterior intracranial optic pathways.
d) Rarely — subdural haematoma if iso-dense with brain tissue on the scan.

7. ISOTOPE BRAIN SCAN

Technetium 99 m is the usual isotope.
May, but does not invariably, demonstrate intracranial neoplasms, e.g. meningiomas, vascular gliomas, metastases.
Poor indication of lesions in the posterior fossa.

8. ARTERIOGRAPHY

Mortality up to 0.25%.
 Carotid, vertebral, or less commonly arch aortogram. Depending on vessel injected, will show intra and extracranial vessels, and presence or absence of:
a) Constriction of vessels.
b) Obstruction, e.g. by embolus.
c) Loss of vascular patterns, e.g. in arterial thrombosis.
d) Displacement, e.g. by space occupying lesions.
e) Pathological circulation in some neoplasms or vascular malformations.
f) Aneurysm formation.
g) Venous thrombosis.

9. X-RAY CONTRAST ENCEPHALOGRAPHY

Using air or myodil. Usually restricted to neurosurgical centres, and now performed after an initial CAT scan.

Neurophysiological investigations

1. ELECTROENCEPHALOGRAPHY (EEG)

Records electrical activity over the brain; usually over the scalp, rarely intracerebral.

a) *Electrodes*: usually 22, placed at uniform intervals, according to the International 10–20 system.

b) *Connections*: bipolar (2 electrodes) or monopolar to a specified reference electrode.

c) *Recording*: eyes open and closed, also 3 minutes hyperventilation, and brief photic stimulation at varying flicker rates.

d) *Activity*:
   Delta: ½–3 Hz (cycles per second)
   Theta: 4–7 Hz
   Alpha: 8–13 Hz
   Beta: 14–30 Hz

e) *Normal activity*: waking record — either alpha posteriorly (amplitude 25–100 microvolts), and beta anteriorly (amplitude approximately 15 μv.), or generalised low amplitude beta.
   Drowsiness — alpha intermittently decreased, theta appears.
   Sleep — delta and some theta activity. Runs of fast activity — sleep spindles, and arousal 'K' complexes.
   Children — varying amounts of slow activity, gradually replaced by alpha with increasing age.

f) *Abnormal activity*:
   1. Reduced amount and amplitude of normal frequencies, and/or excess slow frequencies, can be generalised or localised.
   2. Abnormal waveforms — sharp waves (transient waves of peaked outline, 70–200 milliseconds duration); spikes (duration 20–70 msec.); spike and slow wave complexes, either occurring spontaneously or in response to provocation by hyperventilation, photic stimulation or sleep.

NOTE: (i) A single normal EEG *never excludes* intracranial pathology, but in certain suspected conditions makes the diagnosis *very unlikely*, e.g. cerebral abscess, encephalitis, frequent apparent minor absences.

    (ii) Serial recordings may show deterioration (e.g. with neoplasms) or improvement (e.g. after a cerebrovascular accident), therefore more helpful than a single record.

    (iii) If generalised excess slow activity is seen, need to exclude metabolic causes, e.g. uraemia, electrolyte imbalance, hypoglycaemia, or liver failure before assuming primary intracerebral lesion.

g) *Indications for EEG*
1. Differential diagnosis of episodic loss of consciousness.
2. Differentiation of focal attacks, e.g. temporal lobe epilepsy, focal motor or sensory symptomatic 'partial' epilepsy. Sleep recording can activate temporal lobe foci.
3. Serial assessments in epilepsy, e.g. may reveal developing neoplasm, or chronic degenerative condition. Useful in detailed preoperative assessment. If surgery, e.g. lobectomy, contemplated for intractable fits — bilateral foci a contraindication to surgery.
4. Serial examination helpful in distinguishing neoplasm from vascular lesion, may indicate a need to repeat CAT scan.
5. Investigation of unexplained behaviour disorder in children can reveal undetected minor absences, temporal lobe foci, deteriorating cortical function, e.g. in cerebral degenerative disorders, or indicate possibility of brain damage at birth.
6. Investigation of suspected abscess, can indicate need for CAT scan, e.g. in meningitis without focal signs.
7. Confirmation of brain death. Two *iso-electric* (flat) records, at intervals of 24 hours, using maximum amplification ($10\mu v/cm$). There must be no evidence of hypothermia or barbiturate intoxication, which are potentially reversible causes of a flat record.

h) *The EEG and epilepsy*: an EEG, *during* a major, focal, or minor fit, which shows specific ictal abnormality, *is diagnostic* of an epileptic attack. Conversely a generalised attack without appropriate simultaneous EEG changes indicates that that particular attack is not a genuine fit.

A normal inter ictal EEG does *not* exclude a diagnosis of epilepsy, which is primarily a clinical assessment based on the history and an eye witness account.

An abnormal interictal EEG may, but does not necessarily indicate epilepsy. Generalised, episodic, interictal EEG spike and wave activity, with a history of attacks of loss of consciousness, gives support to a diagnosis of a liability to epilepsy.

Spike and wave EEG activity in response to photic stimulation, the photoconvulsive response — supports a diagnosis of a liability to fits, *but* also occurs in approximately 1% of normal children who never have fits. In psychomotor epilepsy and temporal lobe attacks, a routine and a sleep EEG will reveal spike foci in almost 90% of patients. *N.B.* Useful in assessing cause of episodic aggressive behaviour, but *rarely* of help in deciding if a criminal episode occurred during a fit.

Fit frequency and degree of EEG abnormality *not* closely related in major focal attacks, but definitely related in minor or petit mal attacks.

2. ELECTROMYOGRAPHY (EMG)

Electrical activity in muscles can be recorded over the surface using surface electrodes, or by fine needle electrodes within the muscle itself. All muscle fibres innervated from one anterior horn cell are called a motor unit. The number of fibres per unit varies from 10–12 for ocular muscles to greater than 1000 in gastrocnemius.

The motor action potential is the summated electrical activity from all fibres in one motor unit, of duration 2–10 msecs, amplitude $100\mu v$ to 2 MV.

Relaxed normal muscle is electrically silent, except when needle electrodes are introduced near the motor end plate area, when low amplitude biphasic potentials may be seen.

Abnormal spontaneous activity in resting muscle
a) Fibrillations: brief 0.5–2.0 msecs, low amplitude ($30–150\mu v$) potentials, may be due to endplate activity, and occur pathologically in denervation.
b) Positive sharp waves: low amplitude, may be of longer duration than 10 msecs, occur with local muscle trauma and denervation.
c) Fasciculations: spontaneous, often visible, contraction of groups of muscle fibres or motor units; can occur in healthy muscle, particularly if cold. Usually indicates anterior horn cell damage.
d) Myotonia: high frequency discharge of action potentials, variable frequency 10–150 per sec. Sounds like a 'dive bomber'.

Denervation. Causes loss of motor units, reduced number of action potentials during full voluntary contraction. In chronic denervation with reinnervation, units are of increased amplitude and duration, often polyphasic. Variable irregular recruitment of units during contraction.

Myopathy. Primary muscle diseases — individual units abnormally brief, low amplitude and polyphasic. Initially no obvious loss of units on maximum contraction.

3. NERVE CONDUCTION STUDIES

Conduction velocity can be measured both in motor and sensory nerves. An evoked muscle action potential (MAP) is recorded either by surface or needle electrodes. Stimulation of a motor nerve, usually with a square wave pulse of very brief (0.1–0.5 msecs.) duration; must be supramaximal intensity. Latencies are measured to the onset of the MAP from two separate stimulation points.

$$\text{Conduction Velocity} = \frac{\text{difference in latencies}}{\text{distance between stimulation points}} \text{ (CV)}$$
(expressed as metres per second m/sec)

It is approximately 50 m/sec in the nerves of the arms, 40 m/sec in the nerves of the legs.

The sensory action potential, recorded over or near the nerve, is of lower amplitude than the MAP (approximately 10μv), averaging techniques often required to distinguish the response from background 'noise'.

Axonal damage causes minor abnormality of the CV, but demyelination can reduce the velocity to less than 15 m/sec. The evoked MAP becomes reduced in amplitude, and polyphasic or 'dispersed' due to summation of abnormal later responses. Sensory nerve damage causes reduced amplitude sensory action potentials, when damage affects the primary afferent neurone. Lesions proximal to the sensory ganglia leave distant sensory responses intact.

4. OTHER EVOKED POTENTIALS

a) Visually evoked potentials
Light stimulation causes an evoked response which can be recorded on the scalp over the occipital cortex. Averaging procedures improve the definition of the response. Stimulus may be a flashing light, but response is more uniform with alternating black and white checker board, which is reversed at a rate of 2 per second. The latency between stimulus and response, normally approximately 100 msec, is increased by damage to the optic nerve or intracranial visual pathways.

Optic neuritis causes significant delays in over 90% of patients. In patients with multiple sclerosis, both with and without known previous retrobulbar neuritis, the response is delayed in at least 70%.

b) Auditory evoked potentials
Scalp recordings of electrical responses to auditory stimuli always require averaging techniques for display, as amplitude only 0.5–1μv. Multiphasic responses have been identified and brain stem components delineated. In multiple sclerosis, brain stem components delayed in 46% of patients with appropriate signs, but delays also reported in over 50% of those without brain stem signs. N.B. Other pathological disturbance of brain stem function may also delay the responses.

c) Electrospinogram

Skin surface recordings over the cervical cord region, in response to electrical stimulation of the median nerve yield well defined potentials when averaging techniques employed. If delay in the peripheral nerve component is excluded, then any delay in latency reveals proximal abnormality. Increases have been reported in 64% of patients with multiple sclerosis without clinical signs to suggest cervical cord involvement.

FURTHER READING

Laidlaw, J. & Richens, A. (1976) *A Textbook of Epilepsy*. Edinburgh: Churchill Livingstone.

Lenman, J. A. R. & Ritchie, A. E. (1970) *Clinical Electromyography*. London: Pitman.

McDonald, W. I. & Halliday, A. M. (1977). Diagnosis and classification of multiple sclerosis. *Brit. Med. Bull.*, **33**, 4–8.

5. SOME ABNORMAL EEGs

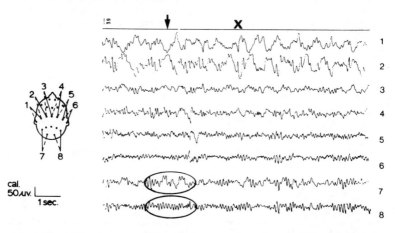

Fig. 1. Female patient, aged 40, with an extensive glioma in the left temporal lobe. The EEG shows localised slow waves over the left temporal area. In channels 1 and 2 there are delta waves and some show phase reversal, (↓) being deflected down in channel 1 and up in channel 2. Occasional single waves of sharp outline also show phase reversal between channels 1 and 2. (×) Alpha activity in channel 7 is less regular than in channel 8, and there are underlying theta and delta waves in channel 7 (◯).

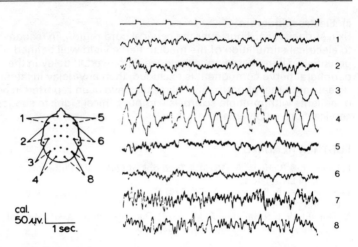

Fig. 2. Child, aged 12, with a right-sided Todd's paralysis. EEG taken two days after the focal fit. Localised left hemisphere slow wave activity is seen in channels 3 and 4. Subsequent investigations failed to reveal any obvious cause for the clinical manifestations. The child made a good recovery and the EEG returned to normal.

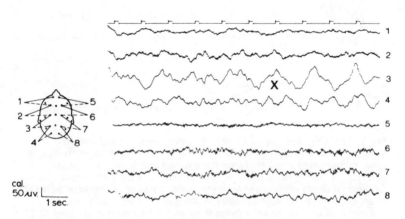

Fig. 3. Child, aged 8 months. Record shows unilateral delta waves (×) over the left hemisphere — especially in channels 3 and 4. This abnormality resulted from a prolonged right-sided fit in a child who had had infantile spasms at age 5 months, but whose CAT scan was normal.

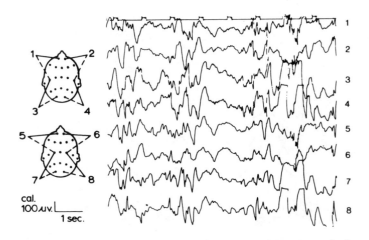

Fig. 4. Child, aged 5 months. Episodic bursts of high amplitude mixed spike and slow waves, separated by periodic suppression of electrical activity. Hypsarrhythmic EEG in a child with salaam spasms.

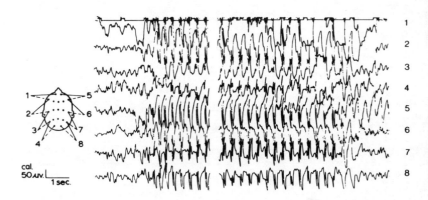

Fig. 5. Child, aged 7 years. Minor absences of petit mal type. EEG shows generalised spike and slow wave complexes starting and ceasing synchronously over all areas, during which the child failed to respond to simple commands.

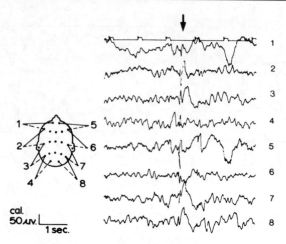

Fig. 6. 7-year-old child with grand mal epilepsy. Bilateral spike and slow wave discharges. Phase reversal of spike and slow wave components seen over both hemispheres, between channels 1 and 3, as well as 4 and 6. (↑)

PART III

On taking examinations

Examination technique and some common faults

This section discusses the faults which are commonly committed by both undergraduate and postgraduate candidates for examinations in psychiatry and suggests ways of avoiding them.

THE PAPERS

Multiple choice
It is important to attempt all the questions and a careful watch on the way you allocate your time is essential. It is never advisable to guess, because you can lose marks for wrong answers. Read the precise wording of each question carefully and allow time to go back over items on which you are not certain.

The essay paper
Again it is crucial that you budget your time efficiently. So often the amount written on successive questions becomes progressively smaller, and the bad candidate may furnish only a few scrappy lines as his last answer, sometimes with naive apologies. It is not possible to gain more than a limited number of marks for long answers but many can be lost through a failure to complete the paper adequately, and with a close marking system this is a most important point to remember.
   A good essay answer should pay attention to the following points:

Legibility, coherence and style
Attention to basic English grammar and care over tidiness and legibility seem obvious points, but they are very frequently ignored. This of course implies a lack of consideration for the examiner, who is then in turn less inclined to give the borderline candidate any benefit of doubt.

Planning
An essay type answer should contain an introduction which sets out the general aims of the answer, a body and it should end with relevant conclusions. By all means use headings but avoid using

long and ill-explained lists. Do not waste time on pointless repetition and recapitulation.

Information
To omit important facts suggests carelessness or ignorance: errors of commission are clearly due to inadequate knowledge of the subject: irrelevance suggests lack of care in reading the question, poor judgement regarding what to include, or 'padding' because of inadequate command of the relevant facts.

The answer should cover all relevant aspects of the topic and it should avoid a too limited approach. For example, discussion of assessment should include special investigations as well as clinical evaluation and differential diagnosis: it may be necessary to refer to all age groups, though not uncommonly either children or adults are discussed as opposed to both.

An unduly restricted interpretation of the question is a very common fault. Another is the failure to include hard facts such as the absolute or relevant incidence of syndromes (for example that Alzheimer's Disease is far more common than Pick's Disease), the incidence of symptoms, or the proportion of patients responding to treatment. All these are relevant to clinical skills and judgement.

Explanation and definition
A poor candidate tends to indulge in the use of technical terms and concepts in a way which does not indicate whether he really understands them. It should be a golden rule that adequate explanation must be provided at all points and the answer should be liberally laced with phrases such as 'by which I mean', or 'by this is meant'. It is not sufficient to take technicalities for granted, assuming that the examiner understands them and that he will necessarily believe that you do too. Whenever a diagnostic entity such as depression is mentioned you should explain what you mean by it. All terms should be used with the utmost care: avoid those such as 'inadequate' or 'psychopathic' unless you are prepared to define them fully. These points are of course particularly important when new concepts such as 'high expressed emotion' or 'face to face contact' are being considered.

Critical and well-reasoned discussion
You should attempt to show that you can think for yourself as opposed to merely reproducing lists obtained from books, and that you can apply in a sensible way the concepts which you discuss in the light of adequate clinical experience and with a correct sense of priorities. Avoid a superficial approach and the use of clichés, for example by describing treatment merely as 'supportive psychotherapy involving a multidisciplinary approach with a social worker seeing the family and occupational therapy'. Each of these needs further explanation and justification. Unsatisfactory essay

answers in clinical psychiatry, even in postgraduate examinations,
are often written at a level which could be produced by a well
informed layman: the combination of superficiality of approach,
failure to define technical terms which are used uncritically, all
contribute to a bad overall effect on the reader. Many of
these errors are due to faulty examination technique and with
adequate practice and preparation they can of course be avoided.

Reference to the clinical situation
In order to demonstrate that you can apply theoretical knowledge
in practice, you should provide an essay answer which contains
adequate reference to the relevant clinical situation. In this way
theoretical issues can be explained more fully by illustrating how
they may be applied.
  You should also demonstrate that your priorities are correct and
that you are able to distinguish between common and rare
conditions, or hazardous from harmless procedures. You should try
to show that you are sufficiently critical of the terms and concepts
which you use by indicating the limitations of their application.

Breadth of approach
Although you may feel a certain partisan allegiance to one or more
theoretical approach, you should do justice to all others which may
be relevant: you must be able to show that you can evaluate a
variety of view points without prejudice. In discussing the causes or
management of any condition make sure that you cover such
aspects as epidemiological, social, psychological and nursing as
well as more obvious clinical problems. Do not forget to consider
differential diagnosis: few psychiatric syndromes are so well
defined that no others are relevant, and take care to discuss all
other possible contenders at all points. Do not deal with diagnostic
categories as if they are disease entities akin to those of general
medicine, but remember that most are loose descriptive
syndromes: the best example of this error is the way reactive and
endogenous depression are so often assumed to be mutually
exclusive without any attempt being made to define the basis for
distinguishing between the two.

Avoidance of other common errors
Do not make silly casual comments. If you bring in your personal
experiences make sure that you do not base your answer entirely
upon them: demonstrate that you also have an adequate
knowledge of the literature and the views of others. If you mention
authors only do so when you can furnish correct details of their
findings otherwise you merely give the impression of 'name
dropping'. Avoid using your answer to indulge your views on
irrelevant general issues such as the state of society or other
organisations and disciplines. Always ask yourself whether these

matters are strictly relevant. Be precise over what you write, avoid unstructured verbosity and take care over how you express your ideas. The candidate who wrote 'criminal shop lifters should be eliminated' produced a rather comic effect which was probably unintended but which did nothing to add to the quality of his answer.

THE CLINICAL

The precise form will of course vary according to the particular examination being taken. The M.R.C.Psych. examination allows the candidate one hour to assess his patient and this is followed by a five minute review period during which he gathers his ideas together before being interviewed by two examiners for a total of 30 minutes on matters relevant to his case.

In most examinations the 'clinical' is regarded as a crucial part of the test and must be passed. Adequate attention to examination strategy is nowhere more important than here.

Patient assessment

In order to work as quickly as possible, a systematic approach to the history and mental state is essential. Always ask whether physical examination is mandatory: usually you will be expected only to carry this out if you think it is relevant to the particular problem with which you are dealing. In any case it is probably advisable to allow the last few minutes or so to check the blood pressure, optic fundi and reflexes, if only rather summarily: sometimes something unexpected and surprising turns up and you will then be likely to earn extra marks. Remember that you can still carry on talking to your patient whilst checking physical signs and so elaborate on gaps in the history if necessary.

The review period

During this time you must assemble the relevant positive points clearly in your mind. A good way of doing this is to prepare a formulation from the notes which you have made during your interview with the patient. In the M.R.C.Psych. examination it is assumed that candidates will have organised their findings and conclusions in this way before they proceed to interview with the examiners. The candidate's task is not made easier by the fact that the term 'formulation' can have a variety of meanings. The following scheme has the advantage that is promotes a comprehensive summary of all the available data. Such an approach is essential in the face of a bewildering variety of information. The proposed formulation (developed by Kräupl Taylor) forces you to commit yourself with regards to what is relevant and to a logical systematic approach. It should also give you confidence because its systematic approach helps you to remember the relevant facts. The candidate who proceeds to meet the examiner without having to search nervously through a mass of notes and one who can speak from memory creates a good impression immediately. Practice at formulation permits this to be done.

An adequate psychiatric formulation has the following headings:
Descriptive: a few sentences summarising the essence of the history and mental state. This should take two or three minutes only.
Diagnostic: your first choice syndrome and you will need to justify it.
Differential diagnostic: the other possibilities with points for and against.
Aetiological: include all types of possible causes.
Psychodynamic: outline any themes which are discernible.
Therapeutic: how you would proceed in management.
Prognostic: what you think the likely outcome will be.

You should take care to consider these aspects of formulation in the above logical sequence because failure to do so leads to confusion. Never consider treatment before summarising the clinical features and diagnosis.

Interview with examiners
To have a systematic and comprehensive formulation allows you confidence when you proceed to your interview with the examiners. At first you may be asked to re-interview your patient very briefly in the presence of the examiners in order to illustrate the main symptoms of mental phenomenon. Your relationship with your patient, your ability to put him at ease and your skill with which you handle a brief yet relevant discussion will be evaluated at this point.

The patient having left, your interview with one of the examiners now begins: the other may ask a few relevant questions himself for a short period later. At this point try to keep certain important strategies in mind.

You can anticipate some predictable opening gambits on the part of the examiner who may say 'tell me about your patient' or 'what is your diagnosis' or 'give me your formulation'. Some candidates react by starting on a long detailed discussion of the case history which includes many irrelevancies, and after 5–10 minutes have to be stopped by the examiner. Such a false start situation is harmful: it puts you off your stride and wastes time in which valuable marks might otherwise have been gained. It is best to anticipate and avoid this kind of difficulty by being explicit about your approach and to warn the examiner in advance how you would like to answer his initial question. For example it might be appropriate in response to

'tell me about your patient' to say 'I would like to answer that by
summarising very briefly the main positive findings on assessment
and then proceed to my formulation under the headings diagnosis,
differential diagnosis, aetiology, psychopathology, therapy and
prognosis.' If a formulation is requested state the seven headings
under which you propose to discuss it. Many candidates are so
anxious that they become over-inclusive: they are afraid to
summarise their findings and opinions and are reluctant to opt for
diagnostic priorities. They clutch their notes nervously and scan the
examiner's face for inspiration. You will appear far more confident
if you are armed with a systematic formulation which allows you to
summarise the facts and to present the case in a fluent and logical
way. So often the examiner is faced with an immensely detailed yet
haphazard account and he has to interrupt repeatedly in a search
for relevant data. The candidate who can proceed logically through
a seven point formulation which has been suggested here cannot
fail to impress.

Be prepared for interruptions and don't be put off by them:
practice being interviewed by your fellow trainees in this way.
Argue your point firmly and try not to shift your ground just to
please the examiner or to sound out his views before starting to
state yours. If you don't know, say so and do not hedge.

Do not look for hidden traps and try to avoid an argument.
Remember that the examiner who seems unduly critical may well
appear so because he thinks you are doing well and so he is trying
to find out the full extent of your knowledge by asking difficult and
exacting questions. Control your own emotional reaction to what
happens in the interview and try to deal with each point
systematically rather than in a haphazard way. As in essay writing,
try to define all the terms you use and do not use them loosely.

THE ORALS

These usually consist of a series of questions covering a wide
range of topics which may or may not be relevant to any speciality
in which you work. Try to provide crisp relevant answers. The best
prepared candidates have usually acquainted themselves with
topics of current interest, for example the recent review of the
Mental Health Act or the College report on ECT, as well as having
scanned the main psychiatric journals for recent reviews and
general articles. Remember that the examiner will want to pass the
candidate who has adequate knowledge, who can evaluate it
critically, and who demonstrates that he has had clinical experience
sufficient to apply it with a good sense of priority and judgement.

In preparing for examinations candidates far too often invest an
excessive amount of their time in learning a very great deal of

small print material from text books. It would be far better if more time was spent in practising case presentation and discussion of basic topics with colleagues or tutors. This of course needs more planning and organisation in one's learning and revision, compared with comfortable arm-chair reading. Such an approach is well worth the effort, however, and will help you to avoid many basic errors which frequently contribute to failure in clinical examinations.

Index